BEATING

THE

BLOWFISH

FOR

My family:
Mummy, Daddy, Rupert and Kate.
Your love and support has been
unconditional and complete.

The boys:
Rich and Loz,
a truly formidable duo.

The girls:
Gail, Rach, Gilly, Jen and Em,
without whom the blowfish
would have remained undetected.
I will be forever grateful for
your dedication and patience.

Beating the Blowfish

A candid account of
a young yacht skipper's
battle with breast cancer

Emma Pontin

SEAFARER BOOKS

SHERIDAN HOUSE

© Emma Pontin 2009

Published in the UK by Seafarer Books Ltd
102 Redwald Road • Rendlesham • Suffolk IP12 2TE
www.seafarerbooks.com

ISBN 978-1-906266-15-8 paperback

British Library Cataloguing in Publication Data:
Pontin, Emma.
Beating the blowfish.
1. Pontin, Emma. 2. Pontin, Emma – Health.
3. Breast – Cancer – Patients – England – Biography.
4. Women sailors – England – Biography.
5. Sailors – England – Biography. 6. Yacht racing.
I. Title
362.1'9699449'0092-dc22
ISBN-13: 9781906266158

Published in the USA by Sheridan House Inc
145 Palisade Street • Dobbs Ferry • NY 10522
www.sheridanhouse.com

ISBN 978-1-57409-294-3 paperback

A catalogue record for this book is available from the Library of Congress

Photographs that are not otherwise credited are from the author's private collection.
In all cases, the photographs are copyright of the copyright-holder.

Drawing of blowfish by Anya Briggs

Design and typesetting:
Louis Mackay / www.louismackaydesign.co.uk

Editing: Hugh Brazier

Text set digitally in Proforma

Printed in Finland by WS Bookwell

Contents

Foreword
by Dee Caffari MBE

When you are a successful London businesswoman and used to being in complete control of everything a career change is one thing, but a battle to save your own life is a whole different ball game.

I first met Emma at an event in St Katherine's Dock, London. She is a stunning, leggy blonde, who holds the focus of most people when they first meet her. People were genuinely captivated by her fun sense of humour and contagious laughter. She was dynamic, full of energy and had a desire to grasp more of what life had to offer. True to form, Emma had made up her mind on a career change and within months her life had been turned around. No longer did her designer wardrobe pace the streets of London. Her sailing clothes walked the dockside in the UK and she bent the ear of anyone who would listen and who would offer advice. I consider myself fortunate to be one of those people she asked advice from. As another female in this male-dominated environment, I felt able to tell her how it was, simply and honestly, and I was able to offer advice to Emma on what the best practice would be for her to advance in her sailing career.

Following my suggestion of sailing as many different boats as possible and gaining experience from as many different skippers as possible, Emma was off sailing and gaining experience every day. Her confidence and ability improved week by week and her qualifications piled higher and higher. Before we knew it Emma was skippering big boats and guiding others.

Never one to be above her station, Emma was aware of limitations but never saw them as a problem. These were just challenges to be overcome. If she required experience she went and found it. A leg of the Global Challenge Race saw Emma learn a great deal about team dynamics and what makes people tick, as well as developing her sailing skills further. Her mind was set on being selected to skipper a round-the-world yacht race but life threw her the curve ball. Months spent in chemotherapy and radiotherapy meant that her dreams were dashed.

The smile never left her face, and I saw her continuing as a training skipper in between hospital sessions for chemotherapy. Her bandana became a trademark. What was originally something she struggled to accept became the focus of her determination. When she felt she could join me for the Race for Life on Southampton Common, I knew then that she was winning the Battle of the Blowfish.

12 July 2008

'I am having a serious sense of humour failure, Emma!'

Stomping out of my bedroom wearing my shoes, underwear and diamond bracelet, I arrive at the top of the stairs, hands on hips, and retort, 'Well Daddy, they can't start without us!'

Unwilling to be hurried on this day of all days. Returning to the bedroom, I look at my dear friend Gilly, who, as my matron of honour, is hoping that I will now stand still long enough for her to zip me into my wedding dress. I frown at her. She just smiles back at me. She continues to dress me, sets my veil, and then bends down and rubs moisturiser into my legs – and promptly sends me off to get married.

At the top of the stairs I catch a look at myself in the mirror and stare myself straight in the eye. Here we go!

Known for his phenomenal punctuality, my father is pacing the floor in the hall as I totter downstairs in my heels, my feet unused to anything other than sea boots or flip-flops. He is struggling to accept the planned late arrival that is expected of a bride, and as his senior daughter finally emerges, ready at last, he looks up at me and smiles. We are about to make an entrance I am sure many believed we would never make.

Today is my wedding day. Dressed in a beautiful handmade ivory gown which hangs straight and hugs my figure until, tucked just under my bottom, a train streams out. A line of tiny little covered buttons follows the shape of the dress, over which hangs a delicate jacket in ivory chiffon. Around my wrist is the stunning diamond bracelet Rich gave me last night to wear today. I am to sparkle.

Staring at myself in the mirror in the hall, trying desperately not to cry, I think back to the wonderful proposal I received.

So excited, and yet I remember being terrified to dream about this day. It all seemed too far away to imagine, and besides, we had to go to hell and back first. I was sure that I would never be lucky enough to feel these incredible emotions, to experience the wonderful moment when I would be able to stand, squeezing my father's hand, at the entrance to the church on my wedding day.

I

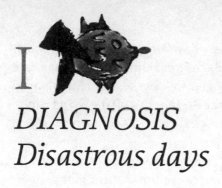

DIAGNOSIS
Disastrous days

July 2006

Life was good. As a professional sailor I had just returned from a fantastic four-month sailing contract on board a Volvo 60, a super-sleek round-the-world racing yacht skippered by a dear friend of mine. We had crossed the Atlantic twice, raced in the Caribbean's premier yacht racing regatta, Antigua Race Week, and competed in the Newport to Bermuda centenary yacht race. It was a lovely hot summer. My boyfriend was due home from skippering a boat in a ten-month round-the-world yacht race, and I was flying out to the penultimate stopover in Jersey to meet him. We had last seen each other three months previously when I flew to Canada from Antigua during a break in my sailing programme. The sun was shining and the world was a wonderful place to be. I was very excited about an energetic future with a man I adored. We are both sailors, and we were planning some time on the water together.

A few years earlier I had given up a successful but more sedentary career in banking law in the City of London, believing there to be more to life than riding the Tube. As a non-sailor I entered a transatlantic yacht race, and after two weeks of sail training I flew to Boston to join my team of thirteen other novices. Our professional skipper and mate were fabulous, relentless and determined, and some thirteen days later we crossed the finish line just off the coast at Southampton in first place. It was a race of challenges for the team, including, for me, a brief unplanned dip in the freezing waters of the Atlantic just off the Grand Banks. However, I had a ball. The real challenge was going to be returning to life behind a desk.

By the summer of 2006 the North Atlantic was no longer an unfamiliar body of water to me. My return to these sunny shores marked my tenth crossing, but I had yet to do so as the skipper. This goal still remained.

On Rich's eventual return to Liverpool in two weeks we were to head off on holiday together to the USA, where I was to meet his three children and finally begin a more traditional period in our new and exciting relationship. We had it all ahead of us. I was fidgety and excitable as I waited at the airport. I did not want this feeling to end.

The feeling *was* sadly to end. Abruptly. My world collapsing in spectacular style.

October 2006

In October 2006 I began what would turn out to be the biggest challenge of my life to date. I am a professional yachtswoman and have raced many oceans the world over, but nothing – *nothing* – could prepare me for what I was about to experience.

A gruelling round of tests and examinations to establish whether the lump in my left breast, the excretion of dark fluid from my left nipple and the large lump under my left arm were the symptoms of breast cancer began after the discovery of a lump in my left nipple in October 2006. Despite the excretion of the dark fluid from my nipple for what was now eighteen months I had not been taken seriously, and tests did not begin in anger until the appearance of the lump.

Previously, back then, I had undergone a breast examination and a mammogram at one of the country's highly respected breast screening clinics in Surrey. I was told that it was duct ectasia – a benign breast disease characterised by the dilation of major ducts within the breast filled with fluid and benign cells. It is a common non-invasive condition that can mimic invasive carcinoma. It occurs traditionally in *older parous* women, and if caught in the early stage it is unlikely to spread outside the breast duct itself.

The treatment for this is an operation to remove the infected ducts. If left unchecked, however, it may develop into invasive breast cancer, and it is this advanced condition that can spread to the rest of the body. If it has spread then the removal of the breast, a mastectomy, is the best and often only form of treatment.

I was advised that I could undergo elective surgery to remove the infected ducts, or alternatively I could choose to live with the nipple discharge, which many women do – apparently! At no point was it mentioned to me that should I choose to leave this situation unchecked there was a risk that it could develop into breast cancer. I elected to have the surgery, but I am ashamed to admit that I am terrified of hospitals and the concept of an anaesthetic horrified me. So when I received the notification of the operation date I wrote to the clinic and raised my fear. They were marvellous and advised me that they would arrange a consultation with an anaesthetist who should be able to put me at my ease. That, sadly was the last I heard from that clinic, and as a result it nearly cost me my life. It was well over a year later, in October 2006, that I eventually found myself attending a different clinic.

Monday 23 October

This morning I attended my final appointment of what is referred to as the Triple Assessment – a systematic three-part method of investigation consisting of a clinical examination, then radiological imaging in the form of a mammogram or a breast ultrasound, then a tissue diagnosis in the form of a fine needle aspiration (FNA) – *a biopsy to you and me* – and finally a core biopsy.

I underwent the mammogram *and* ultrasound, or sonomammogram, followed swiftly by a fine needle aspiration, during which they inserted a needle into the lump with the aim of removing some fluid for analysis. This, I might add, was all done without local anaesthetic – in other words it was agony! But then I am a baby.

By the end of the appointment my poor left breast had been squidged between two rather chilly metal plates into a wholly unnatural shape – flat! – and one I don't believe any boob should be forced into – and had the tiniest of razor-sharp needles inserted into its nipple. Poor little thing!

I drove home to lick my wounds and await my results. I felt uncomfortable and anxious.

I returned to the hospital for the results and they confirmed that whilst they were unable to remove sufficient fluid from my lump there were satisfied that the lump was harmless, a benign cyst, and I should not worry further.

I was delighted by this outcome, and returned home with a spring in my step. I contacted my girlfriends, Em and Gail, and we went out for a glass of wine to celebrate. Clearly everyone had believed it would be cancerous, and the relief on all our faces was evident. I told them the good news, and that whilst the hospital could not extract sufficient fluid, they were sure blah blah blah ... and it was at this point that the girls grabbed me by the hand and said that that was not good enough! I disagreed. I had, sort of, been told that I didn't have a cancerous lump – and that was most definitely *good enough* for me. I argued the toss with them about not needing to go back, but I guess deep down I was wondering, terrified to face the possibility that they might in fact be right. They delivered their big blow, announcing that not only would I need to return but they would be taking me. Basically, they don't believe that I will go!

Monday 30 October

Today one of the girls drove me back to the hospital to undergo a core biopsy. It was truly a mark of her wonderful friendship, love and support that she took the time to drive her terrified friend and her lump into Southampton. Today's activity at least involved a local anaesthetic before I was cut open down the left side of my left breast in an attempt to remove a small section of the lump for further clinical analysis. It was agony once again despite the anaesthetic and I returned home, via the pub, for a large glass of wine.

Scary though it is – do not be put off. Do not be afraid.

Don't sit comfortably in the knowledge that you have had a mammogram and a sonomammogram, when they tell you all is well and that there are no anomalies. The first is considered relatively useless in women under the age of fifty as the tissue is too dense in consistency to read. People are told regularly that they know their bodies better than anyone else, and if that lump that you discover is wrong, then, scary though it is, push for a further examination, a biopsy – anything to further examine what you already know to be unusual.

It might just be that you are the only one in the business of trying to save your life.

Don't be fooled when they say that they were unable to extract sufficient fluid from the lump but they are sure it is just a cyst.

By the time they tell you that the lump under your arm is just a reaction to the needle biopsy your alarm bells should be well and truly ringing.

The simple fact is that if they cannot extract enough fluid it is because there isn't enough fluid in there – meaning that it is not a cyst but cancer!

Hotfoot it down to your local hospital, find your nearest

Australian oncologist and hold on tight! The Aussies are straight-talking and open-minded, and that is what you need by now.

'Hang on,' I hear you say, 'you are marrying an Aussie, you would say that!'

Well yes I am – I am very smart! But he wasn't my oncologist. I don't mean hang on to him that closely! I'm not nuts!

Wednesday 8 November

Departure Day. The excitement around our yacht was wonderful, and for me personally it was magical. I was to skipper this little ship for the first time, from Gibraltar across to the Canary Islands and to the start line of a transatlantic yacht race with my boyfriend, Rich, at my side. Life was good!

The dock was buzzing and my head was deep in the world of weather-routing as I wandered off along the pontoon to consult one final time the various weather websites I had been using to plan our departure and trip. I was to make a decision imminently as to our departure time and, weather permitting, we hoped to leave by mid-morning.

In the event, in a final meeting with the crew I advised them of our plans for an early-afternoon departure. I suggested final shore visits be made and issued an instruction for stowage for sea. Needless to say, as with anything nautical, things took longer than planned, which allowed Rich and me to grab a bite to eat on shore together away from the crew, before slipping lines. We agreed to meet in one of the bars on the marina seafront.

After making our selection for lunch from a rather uninspiring menu we began to discuss the weather and the crossing. My phone rang. It was my parents, wishing us well on our journey.

We continued talking, and then my phone rang again. It was a call that I am sure I will never forget.

After undergoing the raft of tests and examinations a couple of weeks before my scheduled departure to join the yacht in Gibraltar, I telephoned the clinic daily for the results. Conscious of my imminent sailing plans, I was trying to ascertain whether I was fit to travel. I finally received a telephone call from my consultant. He commented that although my results were not back from the laboratory, he had been advised that all was well and he confirmed that he was happy for me to travel. So I packed my bags and flew to Gibraltar.

I was disappointed not to have received the clinical results but was content with my verbal confirmation – although I promised myself that I would call daily from Gibraltar to obtain the exact results.

This I did, and spoke daily with the secretary, each time requesting that the consultant telephone me as soon as he had the results. I knew I would feel happier that way.

Checking the number on the screen, I answered the call with nothing but a passing thought that at least I would set sail with a clean bill of health. I was expecting my consultant surgeon to call, all was to plan.

I moved away from the table so that I could concentrate, and after the standard chitchat the consultant dealt me a blow that I had not prepared myself for.

'The prognosis for you is good, Emma. However, the prognosis for your breast is not. You have a 7 mm grade 3 invasive malignant tumour in your left breast that has spread to your lymph glands, and you should seriously consider having a mastectomy as soon as possible.'

Ending the call and with incredible control I stood and returned to the lunch table. Rich looked at me with a questioning face and I told him my news. 'I have breast cancer,' I said. And then it hit. The reality of what I had been told – the fear, the panic and the clear, but irrational, understanding that I was to die. The tears came flooding and I felt Rich's arms around me

– tight and safe and warm – a place I have always enjoyed being for so many reasons, and I will forever remember that feeling of safety. I buried my head in his chest and he held me close to him. Nothing was said.

After a period of time that felt like an eternity he picked up the phone and telephoned my consultant. A clear and frank discussion ensued between them and plans were made for my immediate return.

During this time I waited, sitting motionless, numb with shock, staring at the yachts in the marina, mesmerised by their familiar shapes and the comforting sound of the rigging. I was thinking about *that* call – remembering my consultant's words: 'Where are you Emma? ... You must be very excited about your race ...'

And yet he knew, he knew I would not be on that race. Why had he asked those questions? My mind was buzzing, filled with questions that had no answers. If we had slipped lines mid-morning as had been the original plan I would have been at sea and would not have received the news, not have received that call, for a further seven days. Would that delay have been too late for me? Too late to save my life? I will never know now.

I recall us speaking about *consideration*. I should *consider* having a mastectomy, he said.

I remember his words clearly, but for me *consider* seemed an odd choice of word. I thought – no, there is no consideration to be made. If this is an operation that will save my life then a mastectomy it must be. Surely a life with one boob would be more fulfilling than dying with two?

My mind raced on. Breast cancer happens to other people, people who are older than me, people who lead unhealthy lives and eat badly, who do little or no exercise. I was surely too young and fit for this. Clearly I was wrong.

My mind jumped continuously and chaotically from one place to the next. I thought about my grandmother and my aunt, both of whom had died of breast cancer. I began to panic. I was going to die too. Everyone did. I couldn't say the words.

Rich's voice interrupted my thoughts and he spoke at length about the phone call and the options available to me. I should undergo this mastectomy as soon as possible, and they presented two dates – next Monday or next Wednesday. The alternative was to wait a further seven days for the operation, by which time Rich would be home with me, but there seemed little point delaying this life-saving operation. I will never forget that moment.

So, sitting at the marina's edge wrapped in Rich's arms with the warm sun on my young body and shaking with fear and being forced to come face to face with my own fragility, I made what, on the surface at least, was a relatively easy decision under the circumstances. I was to fly home immediately and, as advised by my new medical team, was to undergo a mastectomy next Wednesday. For me it was surely the sooner the better. Anything that would give me a better opportunity of surviving was a good thing and should be done immediately.

Things are easy when you have no choice – it is only when you are asked to make a decision that complications and reservations creep in.

Whilst Rich took over my role of skipper and continued to prepare the crew and boat for sea, I spent the afternoon with the parents of some friends of ours who live in Gibraltar and who were simply magnificent. They were strong and reasoned with me but I could hear little as I sat and cried.

I sat at the airport this evening thinking back over the last couple of days and remembering in particular a visit I made to the dentist yesterday. Our friends took me to their dentist – I needed a filling, and a temporary fix would have to do until I returned home. He asked whether I was taking any medication regularly. After my negative response he moved on to ask if I had ever suffered from any of the following conditions: a heart problem, a stroke, diabetes or cancer.

———

Oh God if only I had known! I would be haunted forever by this innocent and apparently harmless conversation with a dentist.

Wednesday 8 November – midnight

I arrived, sombre and tearful, at midnight last night into Gatwick airport on a cold November morning and fell into the arms of my father and my mother. No words were spoken, just hugs and loving faces tinged with terror as we silently acknowledged what was happening.

I sobbed heavily the whole way home whilst Daddy drove through the darkness. Nobody spoke.

We arrived home to carnage. My folks are in the process of completely renovating their home, and there are no interior walls and no roof. They have decamped into my brother's caravan, which they have borrowed and which is temporarily located in their back garden.

Thursday 9 November

This morning was cold and rainy. Last night I slept a fitful sleep – wrapped in a duvet wedged into the converted saloon section of the sitting room area inside a twenty-foot caravan with the rain hammering against the flimsy walls.

I had spent the early hours of the morning awake, thinking, listening to the breathing of my parents asleep in the bedroom of the caravan, my imagination running wild, wondering what the days ahead would hold. Will the team I am to be issued with be more useful than the medical clowns I have to date had the misfortune of meeting?

As dawn broke, Daddy brought me tea and Mummy sat on my makeshift bed with me. We spoke a little, but what could they say to me? This was not supposed to happen!

I watched my mother intently. My eyes studying her face. When I was fourteen years old I had watched her nurse her mother and her sister in our house, both of whom had been diagnosed with breast cancer and died within two years of one another. I wondered what was going through her mind. I felt ashamed and guilty and horrified for her. Whatever her true thoughts this morning she showed me nothing but love.

I have never needed my parents more than I did this morning. At thirty-six years old I turned to them, a helpless child once more, desperately needing their love, encouragement and support – support that no-one else can ever give.

To my delight and surprise Rupert and Kate, my brother and sister, arrived for breakfast ...

... and so the circus began!

I spent an amazing day with my parents, brother and sister, and whilst I remained dazed throughout with red eyes and tears streaming down my face for most of the day, I felt the warmth and support of my family – who generally had no idea really what to say to me. I listened.

A list of questions began – questions that all of us needed answers to. The news had left us completely shell-shocked and devastated but their positive words were encouraging. I don't think that I have ever fully appreciated the amount of love our original unit of five generated.

Sadly Rich was not with us today as he is still at sea, skippering the yacht that I was supposed to. He will return, but only after my mastectomy operation, which is devastating for me.

I wandered off into my own thoughts a lot this afternoon. I had too much time to think, which proved to be a bad thing. My mind just runs wild and my imagination is a very dangerous place at the moment. You see, I am terrified. I am sorry to admit that at this point I am not able to find the strength and drive that everyone would so want me to find to fight this just yet – I am working on that, I promise. I have been searching my soul for the stubbornness and determination that I normally have with everything, and I have resolved to be at that point soon – but I think it is too soon to expect miracles.

To be truthful I feel that I am heading full-speed into a brick wall and I cannot stop the truck – there is no point in holding my foot over the brake pedal – there isn't one! The fear that I have felt this past twenty-four hours has been all-encompassing, and there is nothing, *nothing*, that I can do except lie down and take the hit.

Trying to take stock, I acknowledge that there are many friends and family who will work with me on this challenge – not least the little people, my brother's twins, who, at the age of six, have the biggest role of all – that of making their Auntie Em laugh. They have always been able to do that, and I realise I need that more than anything right now, if only to stop the tears. So many tears. I have been bombarded with love and support from the few friends who know at this stage, and that is over-whelming too.

Rupert told me today that we will win but I cannot see that far yet because I don't know what I am fighting. Kate told me that I am brave because I have faced it head on. I can assure you I don't feel brave. I feel terrified and convinced that it will all go wrong and that the doctors will have more horrific news for me next Thursday when they come and see me after the operation – during which, I have now convinced myself, they will discover that the cancer is everywhere and not just in my breast. My fears are firmly based on the fact that they haven't got any of this right so far. In fact, I remember, they were absolutely clear in their first diagnosis that it was not cancer, and their patronising words of dismissal come flooding back to me.

We agreed as a family to rise to this new challenge and to meet here once more, one year from today, and raise a glass to a successful battle and a healthy future. I was unconvinced, and by no means as optimistic as everyone else about this commitment, but I reluctantly confirmed that I would be there.

Friday 10 November

I returned home early last night, back to Hamble, to face reality. Kate drove me and we talked non-stop all the way. I expressed my need to 'see' this thing, this invisible monster that was trying to kill me. I had a need to focus on it and to make it real before I could really understand how to fight it. We created a series of various images and pictures before finally coming up with a blowfish – my cancer today became a blowfish. A blowfish is an ugly, spiny, evil, poisonous and wholly unpredictable sea creature that lurks, very quietly and unassumingly, in a little dark corner until POOF! – it puffs up into a ball, exploding, releasing its poisonous spines – and there he sits – well, that is my vision of it anyway, and it was working for me as a focus. I was all of a sudden able to imagine a picture – a creature with eyes that watch me whilst I am incubating it in the warmth and safety of my body, protected, whilst I feed it and make it bigger and stronger. I began to hate it immediately.

I reason that the mastectomy will remove my blowfish (and quite frankly that cannot come soon enough now) whilst the chemotherapy and radiotherapy that follow are tasked to round up those poisonous little spines, or cancerous cells, that are potentially lurking in every corner of my body – waiting!

Now I am able to *see* what I am to fight I feel that it is all a little more manageable. Does any of this make sense? Probably not, but it does to me.

At the risk of sounding like a child – it all just seems so unfair!

I wrote a note to some of my friends this morning. It is a very difficult thing to talk about but I have this news that I want to share with some of them, with the people who mean so much to me. I told them that this week I had been diagnosed with breast cancer and that I am to undergo a mastectomy next week. I told them of the effect the news had had on me and my family. I hoped they would be able to support us.

Re-reading the words, it does not seem real. I am sitting in my dressing gown on our sofa with tears pouring down my face, and as I look down I can see my left boob, the object that is causing such emotional upheaval.

We have a housemate at the moment, Loz, one of my dearest friends, and last night he was a star. For one brief moment, when he took me to the pub whilst supper was cooking at home, life felt normal – it was lovely.

Life won't feel like that for a long time, and that is horrible. In his determination to drive me on he did give me a small goal to work towards, and that is a weekend on the water in January with friends – something I love with people I love. Any other suggestions helping me to get through this nightmare would have been gratefully appreciated. What I really need is a miracle, but that isn't going to happen. I am clearly going to have to face this.

It is time for bed but my mind is full. For my friends who know me well I know I can be a prima donna, but I never wanted to take centre stage like this. I will find this fight, I promise you all.

Sunday 12 November

Life continues in a daze. Yesterday I drove up to see my brother – a weekend with the family – full of the normal things that I am so desperate to cling to.

I am not sure that I should have undertaken a three-hour car journey, as my mind is spinning all the time. I have already competed with millions to get where I am today, I have fought a battle to survive from the minute I was conceived, and I am not about to back down from this battle – I want to survive – again. I want to live my life. I want to grow old disgracefully, and I have to admit that I believe I have found the man I want to do that with.

It is with these thoughts racing through my head that I realise my determination to beat my blowfish – but I don't appear to have managed to convince my soul of that.

I returned this evening to find that miracles do in fact happen – in my absence this weekend my dear friend and long-suffering housemate has managed to learn how to hang the shower mat up without being asked. Something is getting through!

Monday 13 November

Today was the first day of months filled with hospital appointments, and I will always remember today very, very well.

This morning I sat with my mother in a small featureless white room in the 'Chest Department' at the Royal South Hants Hospital in Southampton where I would undergo my mastectomy in two days' time. Previously I had requested a meeting with my consultant breast surgeon to discuss, face to face, the fiasco to date regarding my missed diagnosis and to begin discussions on a more positive note in an attempt to move forward. I wanted to talk about my prognosis and the subsequent treatment. However, he was unavailable and we were met by his colleague, a breast reconstruction registrar.

We began, and the registrar seemed surprised that I was angry and was stunningly rude to me. My mother tried desperately to encourage me to move on to more positive thoughts (I think she was finding it all a little embarrassing) but I knew that I would be unable to move on without answers – an admission from someone, *anyone*, in this team that they had seriously screwed up would be a start. My mother observed that it was only because I have two phenomenal friends who forced me back into hospital to have more, and this time conclusive, tests at the beginning of this nightmare that we were sitting here at all.

I needed to hear the reasons for their actions, or lack of actions, explained. How was it that I could pass under the noses of three different breast medical professionals, undergo the well-known and commonly used 'Triple Assessment' test and fail to be properly diagnosed, despite my familial history? Why the presence of the brown, almost bloody, coloured fluid seeping from my left nipple for the past eighteen months, coupled with the lump in my left breast and the discovery of a large lump under my left arm, failed to arouse their concerns I do not know. Why was the lump that was discovered under my arm attributed to the fact that my lymph system was reacting and 'protecting' my body from the intrusion of the needle during the previous fine needle and core biopsies?

Had they made the assumption that most lumps found in younger women were benign? Were they playing with my life?

Finally, today I did receive an admission of failure, an admission that they had in fact missed the diagnosis, and that sending me off to sea without conclusive results was in fact foolhardy. And with this we moved on.

We discussed at length my mastectomy and the process for Wednesday, who would be in the operating theatre with me and how long the procedure would take – and for the record it only takes a stunningly short forty minutes to completely remove a breast and the lymph glands located under the arm – a process that would be vital with my invasive breast cancer.

After a good hour of discussions, coupled with satisfactory answers, it was in trepidation but with resignation that, with both feet dangling in the paddling pool of hope, I wiped my bloodshot eyes, washed my tear-stained face and dived in.

After all, attitude is everything!

I had always taken my boobs for granted, right up to the point when I was told that they were going to take one away. Whilst I appreciate that a woman is not defined by her breasts, they do contribute to helping a woman feel like a woman.

Wednesday 15 November

They removed my left boob today.

I sat and waited this morning in my sitting room. Alone. Thinking. It was a very bad place to be at this time. I should never have been left on my own at this crucial time.

This cancer nightmare was overwhelming on its own, but this was also the first time I had ever been into hospital. My mind destroyed me but I shed no tears.

My parents arrived at 10 am to take me to the hospital but they were early so we sat in silence and waited. After a while I suggested we leave – just listening to the clock ticking until midday would drive me crazy.

I perched on a bed in a ward, the wrong bed as it turned out, and a variety of people were milling around, all in for surgery and all in for different operations, but all of whom were staying just the one night.

My father sat holding my hand. I remember him squeezing the life out of it because it hurt! I remember his strength and support. The doctor came, drew back my gown to reveal my left shoulder and drew a large X on my skin in black ink. 'Don't want to take the wrong breast off now, do we!' he said cheerily to the two of us. I sat in horror – and ricocheting around in my head were the flippant words of a medico who clearly had no understanding of what constitutes fear, words that were thoughtless at a time when I was at my most vulnerable.

For a man who has spent his life 'fixing' me, looking out for me and loving me regardless – rocking me to sleep as I cried, wiping my eyes when I was hurt, cleaning my knees when I fell, helping me with my homework, turning out at all hours to collect me from a pub or party, lending me money when I had miscalculated, putting a smile back on my face – Daddy stood, desperately wishing he could take me away from all of this. As I looked to him my eyes sought his, desperately searching, seeking his help, pleading, now was the time for him to do his stuff, to help me

– and there was simply nothing he could do but watch and hold his little girl as she cried until she lost consciousness.

This cancer has broken the mould. For the first time in his life my father has not been able to 'fix' me.

When I awoke I remember my family standing beside my bed and the most enormous bouquet of flowers – yellow roses! I knew they were from Rich – they are my favourite! My brother, squeezing my right hand, whispered to me that there was a phone call. I could hear Rich's voice, and his soft words were magical. I tried to respond and my slow sluggish voice muttered the words 'I love you,' but that was all I could manage.

All of a sudden I remember feeling alone. My family had gone and I lay in my hospital bed – a mixture of emotions taking hold – relieved to be alive and through this first part of my nightmare but terrified of the future. The ward was silent and I felt very alone. I drifted in and out of sleep and at 3 am I sent a text to Loz, who was at home asleep – or not! He texted back, 'Legs, what are you doing awake?' ('Legs' is my nickname, a reference to my ridiculously long legs.) It was great to chat.

Thursday 16 November

I remember looking down at my toes – the nails no longer painted red, as they have been since I was about twelve years old. The nail polish had to be removed for my operation, and that tiny change bothered me. Everything was different now – and things were about to get worse.

I returned home to an 'invitation' from my local doctor's surgery to pop in for a smear test – lovely! Just what a girl needs after having a boob removed. Why not – get the remaining part of my femininity violated too – brilliant!

Surely my mastectomy is all over my files and a little bit of diplomacy might be in order – have I not earned a short spell in the prod-free ward? Perhaps I might be permitted to deal with one form of cancer before we consider the chances of having a different type.

In the kitchen was a beautiful basket of ... tomatoes! I am told they are one of the best ways of consuming antioxidants naturally and they were yummy. Loz was a welcome sight and an absolute star. Once I was settled on the sofa, the fussing began. He gave me, in his naivety, a bell! It was nothing short of understated brilliance and yet I suspect he had no idea what he had set himself up for.

Yesterday was a day that we will choose not to dwell on in months to come, a day we will, I am sure, try desperately to forget – probably the most horrific day of all.

Friday 17 November

The phone calls began this morning from my brother. He promised he would call me every night and every morning. I had little to say this morning, just tears as he spoke. His lovely familiar voice telling me that I shall be fine, that we can do this, that I have been his sister all his life so far and that he was not prepared to live any part of his life without me in it and that I still had a part to play. They were such wonderful and special words from the most amazing brother. I knew then that he would keep his promise, he would call me every night and every morning.

I clicked the phone down and then – a moment of silence – no-one in the room with me, no phone, just time to think.

***

Before this fiasco I was offered a job – back on a fleet of large round-the-world racing yachts which is to begin next spring – 12 February, to be precise. The water is where I feel alive, and under normal circumstances that date would just roll around after an exciting winter season in the sun.

However, my world is different now. The sea seems so impossible on this November day, but it's where I want to be right now – at sea, away from this attention, this fussing, the fear of dying, the horror of the situation. Like a child I want to run away to sea and then it will all go away!

I resolved then to make that date – 12 February 2007 – to reach it and not give in to this all-consuming overpowering fear. It fast became my focus, the light at the end of what was to be a very long dark tunnel through the heavy months of our British winter. A reflection of where I wanted to be.

I had a visitor this evening too – a friend of mine who has been through cancer himself and someone who truly understood. Someone who understood what it was like to be told that you have cancer – a sentence I wish on nobody. It was great to see him and to talk, but equally I didn't want to hear his answers, as they scared me. He is fast becoming a focus for me, as he had set his sights on a huge sailing challenge and despite his cancer he achieved his goal. I begin to believe that I can do that too.

Saturday 18 November

Rich returned home in the early hours of this morning. I lay still in our bed, flat on my back and unable to move because of the drains. Tears rolled down my face as I waited to see Rich for the first time since my mastectomy and I had no idea how he would react. After all, I had changed somewhat since he last saw me.

I heard the key in the lock and the door open and close almost silently. He shot upstairs, his footsteps heavy, and stood in the doorway of our bedroom. He looked at me. I noticed how gently he sat down on the bed – in case of breaking me, as if I was made of china. We said nothing to each other. I felt his arms hold me as close as he dared without hurting me. The silence was deafening. There was nothing to say. His eyes were full of love and pain. He eventually slid into bed beside me and snuggled up as close as possible, and his warmth and presence seemed to make it all seem bearable but very, very real. His face told a thousand stories – I wondered what was going through his mind.

It has been a day of many emotions. After that precious and tender reunion in the early hours my family arrived. I found this very hard. I was desperate to see them all but life is different now. I found myself looking at the shape of my mother and Leanne, my sister-in-law, and then glancing down at my now very odd-shaped and lopsided chest and I left the room in tears. I wanted to hide my deformed frame. I shot into the bathroom and took a long hard stare at myself in the mirror. Why me? The tears rolled down my cheeks as I stared at myself. I looked down at my drain sack stuffed into a cloth bag covered in pink flowers that I had to carry around. The other end of the drain was still sewn into my chest, the whole thing was unbearable. How would I ever get through this? I could hear my family downstairs chatting, discussing whether they should come up and check on me. The decision was to leave me for a moment – then 'No, I'll go.' They didn't know what to do for the best, and neither did I.

After a fantastic lunch surrounded by the familiar chaos and bedlam of a Pontin family gathering, engulfed in the warmth and love of my family, we took a slow gentle stroll along to our beach. I needed fresh air but couldn't walk very far. My niece and nephew, twins aged six, held my hand so gently, just like Rich had this morning, as if I was made of china. They smiled and hugged me as we walked.

The troops departed and Rich and I were left alone once more. It must have been difficult for them all today to see me as I was. Not knowing what to expect, how I would react, how I was going to handle the day and quite importantly how they should treat me. It is hard enough for me to take on board, let alone the team that are meant to be supporting me.

Should they smile? Should they talk honestly or factually at the risk of scaring me? Would I be ready to talk about any of it at this early stage? Questions that must have gone through their heads, and that have probably been discussed at great length behind my back so a united and supportive front is presented. Well, they were fantastic. My family knew just what I had wanted, and that was normality, and that is exactly what I got.

Thank you – a truly challenging day for us all. I need a cuddle tonight!

Monday 20 November

Cancer doesn't have a heart – it doesn't listen to us talk, it cannot hear our prayers. I would just like the chance to grow old with Rich, and I will not know if this is possible for another nine days. Will I ever be able to stroll, wrinkly hand in wrinkly hand, along the beach with my beautiful boy? We shall never know, but I would desperately like the opportunity to try. I would like to reward his commitment to me by being there for him.

I have caught him watching me – day in day out – and I often wonder what he really thinks. Does he worry that I won't be here at Christmas despite the fact that he tells me he thinks of our future together, the forty years that we have often promised each other?

Does he wonder why on earth he took this on? Was there an easier option? Yes, of course there was, but that apparently didn't make him very happy.

I braved it today and asked him – why? Why have you chosen to stay? Because of the reaction that you would receive should you cut and run now, or simply because you love me and leaving is not an option?

Simple Em – 'I adore you.' 'You make me complete.'

I knew then for certain that Rich would stand beside me and help me battle through this nightmare and I was grateful. I felt elated and completely and utterly content.

Wednesday 22 November

It is one week on and never have I so desperately wished that I had two boobs! Certain things are meant to be in pairs: legs, arms, eyes, ears and boobs! I am finding it impossible to glance down at my chest. I undress myself with my head held high, not daring to lower my eyes – my form repulses me, and I wonder if that feeling will ever change. The drains have been removed now but there remain in my chest a couple of tiny holes where they once sat.

My mind drifted to my first day home. It was the Thursday, the 'tomato' day. I was bandaged to the hilt with all sorts of padding. I had learned to accept the drain sack that was sewn into my chest and which I carried around stuffed into that pretty little pink drawstring bag made by some ladies at the hospital, which hung from my belt for ease. I remember clearly not being able, or willing, to undress myself, but with the love and support of a girlfriend who came and undressed me I was put in my pyjamas. I sat motionless on my bed staring into her eyes seeking strength, whilst she gently – very gently – removed my top, and feeling, for all the world, like a little helpless child.

As I write this the tears come again. It is only week one for heaven's sake and I have been crying non-stop. So many more tears to shed – but I am exhausted already.

Friday 24 November

Each day my body changes and adapts to its assault – the nerves and skin trying to return to life and accommodate the attack. My chest is tender and I feel like the skin under my left arm has been sunburnt as it is delicate, raw almost, and very tight. The bruising down my left side is very pretty though!

Saturday 25 November

The herculean effort of my family and friends to ensure that I am never alone is amazing. They know that time alone at this stage means time to think and that is dangerous for me.

My heart goes out to Loz really. Friends and family come and visit and I tell them how I am feeling, the same feelings and stories are told over and over again. It must be so totally frustrating to hear the same old anecdotes, but he says nothing.

I made a terrible error today. I caught sight of my operation site this morning – a total and disastrous mistake. I am clearly not able to handle that harsh reality at this point. I have, for want of a better description, been butchered. I realise that it is for my own benefit, for the chance to live, but I look horrific! My boobs represented my femininity and now I only have one. I am no longer the woman I used to be. How am I ever going to face myself, my life and Rich like this. How long will it be before I can look like a woman again?

As usual I turned to my brother, and after a tearful and enormously emotional phone call containing all sorts of meaningful words of encouragement it was concluded that I looked like this because I had apparently chosen life! I just hope that I will be rewarded with life.

Wednesday 29 November

A fortnight of readjustment has passed since I donated my left boob to medical science at the hospital, and I continue to cry and laugh with regular monotony.

Today Rich, my parents and I returned to the hospital for a meeting with my surgeon to receive the results of my mastectomy operation. In abject fear, the likes of which I have never experienced in my life (and would wish on no-one), Rich and I sat in silence staring at the same white walls of that small soulless box room where I had undergone my core biopsy, my heart in my mouth, awaiting the (late) arrival of my surgeon. My parents remained in the huge waiting room whilst we tackled this first stage alone.

The news was good! I was advised that I no longer had a life-threatening disease – a phrase my parents have grabbed hold of with both hands and run with and yet it is not sinking in for me, basically because I simply don't believe them. I know I should and I desperately want to but I am afraid to! I am afraid to get up and fight because I can't handle being knocked back down if they have it wrong – *again*! You see, my thinking is that they cannot knock you down if you are already down. Does that make sense?

Rich wandered off to get my parents, leaving me alone with my thoughts. They returned for the second part of the consultation: the onward treatment.

At this point I was introduced to my oncologist, Dr Peter Symonds, who is an Australian, much to Rich's delight, and a man who I very much hope will help me navigate my way through the next few months.

After introducing himself to me, Rich and my parents he turned his attention back to me and looked me straight in the eye and asked, 'What do you want to do, Emma?' I told him that I wanted to grow old with this man, squeezing Rich's knee. He smiled at me and I knew at that moment, in my heart of hearts, what I had to do, and that I was ready to let battle with my blowfish begin.

I remember very clearly the line that was delivered so precisely. I was told that I no longer had breast cancer (but then I reasoned that I no longer had a breast to have breast cancer in!). The removal of the boob has resulted in the successful slaying of my blowfish, although of the thirteen lymph glands they also removed at the same time four were cancerous. However, I am delighted to report that the cancer has not been found in my bloodstream and is therefore not being delivered first-class to every vital organ in my body. So there is good news in amongst this nightmare, I guess.

I was advised, however, that they will be pumping me full of toxic chemotherapy chemicals for five months, followed by a particularly unpleasant course of radiotherapy, targeting the exact spot on the left side of my chest where the tumours were found in an attempt to chase any little spines down and zap them. Throughout this delightful period of my life I shall take on the appearance of a white snooker ball, and I have been advised that the returning hair may in fact be curly!

I was then advised that there will be a period of recovery before I will be offered the opportunity to undergo reconstructive surgery to include a prophylactic mastectomy and bilateral latissimus dorsi silicone reconstruction.

It appears that at the end of all this I will look more like Pamela Anderson than even I had ever imagined possible – with blonde flowing curly locks and huge silicone airbags.

Speaking of airbags – I have to admit with some reluctance that I have developed a very bad habit, an unhealthy obsession. I have noticed that in my desperate state as the mono-boob resident of Hamble I have spent much of this week gazing longingly at the cleavages of other women. It is a healthy craving to have two boobs I guess. However, I must address this before I find myself with a large black eye.

I have also developed a particularly embarrassing case of nipple envy, and I am embarrassed to admit that I have found myself looking with deep envy at Rich's left nipple.

Thursday 30 November

Today was a day for reflection and too much thought. I am delighted to report, however, that I am at least mobile once more (and not, as it has been suggested, in ever-decreasing anticlockwise circles due to my lopsidedness). This is wonderful after a particularly intense and desperate bout of cabin fever.

On my return home from hospital two weeks ago I was advised by the doctors that I should embark on an extended stay on the sofa to give my body a chance to recover in preparation for the commencement of the chemotherapy. Well for those who know me it will not come as a surprise to learn that I developed a frustrating whinging noise during that time that simply wouldn't clear up! I moaned about having to sit still a lot.

You may remember the issue of a bell. Whilst I appreciate the good intentions with which it was given by Loz in an effort to reduce my wanderings from the sofa – how silly was that! And yes, I know what you are thinking and yes, I did! I abused it out of sheer boredom every now and then and just for a little entertainment value until Rich removed the clapper. How rude!

Needless to say I have not been a particularly well-behaved or stationary patient to date and have driven the boys slowly up the wall. Rich's return on day two proved very helpful to Loz but it meant that I was increasingly restricted in my ability to get away with murder.

So, bell-less, I continue once more to focus on beating this thing.

Anyway, I have been told today that I can be back on the water when I am feeling able (which for my sanity, and that of the boys for that matter, is about now). However, I have been advised that I should not try and cross an ocean single-handed just yet.

Saturday 2 December

Just waiting for your body to fall apart around you – watching, waiting, daily for that difference that shows you are losing the battle.

- Every fifteen minutes someone is diagnosed with breast cancer.

- Eight out of ten women survive breast cancer, but only for ten years.

I have spent much time since my diagnosis considering these facts, facts that are thrown in our faces to highlight the severity of this disease and to encourage us all to fight.

My mind wandered to my grandmother and my aunt once again – two wonderful people who did not beat their blowfish successfully. Two people I miss terribly and two people I would have loved to have had in my life as I grew up, who were taken from me by this disease – and yet I am frightened sometimes to even think about them because I am frightened of failing too. I hate that I often choose to shut out of my mind two such wonderful people but I just have to sometimes – just to get by.

Rich tells me daily, 'You are sparkling, darling! Your eyes are sparkling!' My eyes are his way of judging my sickness or ability to fight this. They are his gauge. I thank heaven that we are all different. I am told time and time again by him that I am still beautiful, and yet I don't feel beautiful – I feel like a freak and it is only going to get worse once the chemicals begin, and I don't think anyone can really understand that.

This evening we sat motionless together on the sofa wrapped in each other's arms engrossed in our own thoughts. The silence was deafening – you could hear a pin drop. The tears rolled down my face once more – God I am tired of crying – it is exhausting but the tears just keep coming ... and it is all only just beginning.

Wednesday 6 December

It has been four weeks since the bottom fell out of my world, three weeks since the mastectomy, and one week since I received the news of my future.

I am struggling today as I consider all that has happened in only four weeks. I have received copious amounts of flowers and cards, letters of support and gifts – all different and all showing each individual's personal approach to handling this mess. I am so grateful for all the notes of encouragement, love and support.

Every time I hear from someone I resolve to find the strength to fight this, the strength that everyone believes that I have. They clearly all know me very well and are the first to admit that I can be an incredibly stubborn and strong-minded individual, but the strength I need for this is herculean and I am really struggling to find it right now – so each note of encouragement makes me feel just a little bit guilty that I am failing, and that pushes me forward.

Rich noted today that whilst he was not sure that I was aware of it, I was reluctant to discuss my cancer in the early days, but he noticed that I searched the World Wide Web in a desperate attempt to learn more about it. It was as if talking about it made it real and reading about it didn't, and I had clearly chosen to read. This would change, he was sure, as the only way to handle an illness such as this was to talk about it and not hide away, imagining that it is not there.

One day, perhaps.

Friday 8 December

I went down to our local pub this evening – braving the world outside the front door. To date the beach had been the only place I had visited as there was no-one there except Rich and me.

Dressed in loose-fitting clothes to hide my deformed shape, we drove into the village and met a couple of friends for a glass of wine. A friend of ours works behind the bar. She was unaware of my 'change in fortune' as someone has put it. I spoke at great length with her in private and discovered that she too had been through cancer – a different form, but she nevertheless understood the rigours of chemotherapy and appreciated my fears.

I smiled. I had known her for a couple of years and knew nothing of her illness. She gave me hope. She was alive, well – very well – and living life to the full. I watched her during the evening and thought – I can do that too!

Monday 11 December

I studied myself in the mirror today – just brave enough to face the reality that is now my life. I stared at my lopsided chest. I looked horrible.

It is very traumatic having a boob removed, but I acknowledge that if I had kept the thing then I would likely have died. I firmly accepted that thought today and finally saw my body as a work-in-progress, a jigsaw that will remain incomplete until I undergo my reconstruction. This has made the whole one-boob issue just a little more bearable.

Thursday 21 December

It has been a pretty uneventful month waiting. I feel like we are treading water. I cannot begin my chemotherapy until the middle of January as they like to give the body eight weeks or so to recover and adjust from the shock of an operation, but I have found this time incredibly frustrating. Having developed a deep hatred for this blowfish I now want to get on with it! Come on! We have come this far – let's keep going.

I began a big challenge this week as Rich returned from the USA with his children this morning. They are staying with us for Christmas, which will be brilliant but quite challenging. I barely know them, having met them once, or is it twice, before. I am keen to get to know them obviously as they are a huge part of the man I love but I am not sure I am up for the job just at the moment. I have not mentioned this to Rich as he is incredibly excited and I don't want to dampen his excitement. I wondered perhaps if their visit should have been postponed but I guess it is an attempt by us both to hold on to some kind of sense of normality.

They arrived bristling with excitement. It was as if a whirlwind had landed – bags and clothes, toys and people everywhere – it was great. They are fabulous children. We have decided not to say anything to them about my cancer until the end of their visit.

Today was emotional for us both but for very different reasons.

Monday 25 December

With every black moment comes a lovely sparkly one too!

Not content with just taking on breast cancer I have now decided that I need a second, more challenging task to go with it and have, in a moment of madness, decided to take on marriage too. In my wisdom I said 'I will' to a wonderful, romantic – and surprising – marriage proposal today.

I sat on the sofa at my parents' home with Rich beside me and opened a large box I had received from him, inside which was a note and another box. After reading the note I opened the next box, which contained yet another note from him. This continued until I reached a note that quite simply took my breath away – in fact it silenced me for a truly amazing and previously unrecorded eight minutes, during which time Rich had slid off the sofa and, unnoticed by me, was on one knee clutching a small blue box containing the most beautiful engagement ring.

Tears rolled down my cheeks, and in the heavy silence Rich asked, 'Shall I take this silence as a yes, then?' As the silence broke my father, who had been privy to the whole plan, having been asked for my hand by Rich in November, produced a large bottle of pink champagne. Oh, and the telephone. My siblings needed to be contacted with this news.

And yes, I know he is Australian, but you cannot have it all!

My brother, when he finally stopped crying – probably over the fact that I am about to give him an Australian for a brother-in-law – seemed delighted to have me off his hands – at thirty-six years old I think he was worried that I would remain his responsibility forever.

My sister, however, should she come down from her mountain explorations in New Zealand, where she has taken refuge this festive period, has yet to discover that she and her bottom, in the role of bridesmaid, have a date with a very large pink bow. On second thoughts, perhaps she should remain there. She never did suit pink!

As the champagne flowed, and with an excitement I almost could not contain, I shot off to call my best friend Gilly. She is a truly special person with whom I have shared everything since we met aged thirteen in the south of France when our families were on holiday. Gilly lives in the Lake District, miles from me, but the distance has never dampened our friendship. She could hear the excitement in my voice bubbling over as I delivered my news.

After minutes of giggles and fidgety excitement discussing the proposal, the ring, colours for the bridesmaids and other girly stuff there followed tears of sadness like no other. My mother popped her head into the library where I was on the telephone and mouthed a message to me. I fell hard onto the sofa as it quickly dawned on me that I had, in the carnage of the last eight weeks, omitted to share with my dearest friend the most devastating news I have ever had the misfortune to share. I drew in a labouring breath and whispered into the phone that I had breast cancer. Her silence was deafening. I could almost hear her tears falling as she spoke gently. I could barely hear her voice asking me why? Why had I not told her? How?

I was aware that I had delivered some horrible news to her and that my timing was rubbish, but we spoke for half an hour or more before we were interrupted and taken back to our respective families. We celebrated my engagement, but my mind was still with Gilly.

I went to bed tonight wondering if I would ever make my wedding day. It should be the most amazing day, when every girl wants to look and feel like a princess, and it was finally on the horizon and yet I had no idea if I would be attending mine – there was so much to go through, so much uncertainty. It could be the light at the end of a very dark tunnel or it could be a dream.

I decided small steps were the way forward. The first tiny step was to make my first chemotherapy appointment, next was to skipper the transatlantic yacht race that was taken from me and then, *then*, the wedding day. Our wedding day. I snuggled deeper into the warm embrace of my fiancé – a man who has never doubted my ability to fight this, a man whose faith in our future has never wavered.

Tuesday 26 December

I thought back on the events of yesterday. How ironic it was that I had purchased for my mother a pair of pink ribbon cufflinks for her to wear in her smart white shirt. They were meant as a symbol of support for the continued research into a disease that had so cruelly taken her mother and her sister. It was ironic as I was unaware that I had breast cancer at the time I purchased them. When she opened the little box wrapped in jolly Christmas paper she looked at me, assuming I had done it deliberately – not so.

I have spent much of today fiddling with my left hand, staring at the rock sitting on my finger. Needless to say I am eager to show off the 'carat' that is making my left hand so incredibly heavy so we (that is, my husband-to-be and I) will be organising an appropriately social function for viewings. As this will be the last time I venture out for some months with a full head of hair, I think it is important that we celebrate!

Friday 29 December

The prospect of having a child is an exciting one for many women. It is simply a case of 'when', but when the possibility of that option is potentially removed panic takes over. At least it does if you are me and fighting a disease that could stop that.

I had assumed like so many women that I would have children at some point and it was just a case of finding the man I adored to share that excitement, responsibility and challenge with. Well, I have now found him and whilst I accept that I have a challenge on my hands with breast cancer I did at least think that perhaps, one day, should I beat my blowfish, we would go on to have a family.

But life is not that simple in the world of chemotherapy and hormone drugs. You see, I have been advised that after chemotherapy and radiotherapy I will then have to go on a five-year course of tamoxifen – a drug that suppresses the production of oestrogen in my body and could basically bring on the menopause. Not great for someone who wants to have children. However, I have also been advised that I would be at risk if I were to become pregnant due to the higher levels of oestrogen in a pregnant woman – the very oestrogen that had contributed to my breast cancer.

I was told quite clearly that Rich did not want to have a child with me at the expense of the life of the mother.

The options available are apparently numerous, but all come with their risks.

Fertility treatment is clearly the most obvious option, and the urgency to harvest my eggs came to light. We would have to delay the start of my chemotherapy in order for the clinic to have time to harvest my eggs otherwise we would have to wait until the end of all of this which might be too late as the tamoxifen might by then have brought on the menopause and an end to that option.

However, this proves risky too as fertility treatment involves pumping me full of oestrogen to help me produce more eggs, thus potentially feeding any leftover 'spines' from my blowfish and potentially making my situation worse.

The question was, did we really want a baby naturally at the cost of my life?

The answer was simple. Chemotherapy! Now!

Saturday 30 December

I find myself watching Han, Dan and Nick – thinking about being their stepmother, wondering if I will ever have any children of my own. They are delightful children and I love their company but I have never thought about being a stepmother. I wonder what they think of me. Too scared to ask just yet.

Sunday 31 December

Unsurprisingly, I spend many hours asking 'Why me?' Is this punishment for something I did? Did I lie as a child, should I not have hit my brother in the face when I was eight, was I not supposed to resent the arrival of my wee sister because she was too cute and it took the attention away from me, was I not supposed to have worn leg warmers with my ra-ra skirt, should I have finished what I started when I went into law and not left when I discovered something much more fun? The truth is I am never going to know why, but I keep asking, and I will keep asking until I reach peace with myself and accept that there is no answer to that question.

We trundled up to Woodford today to see in the New Year with my brother and his family full of positive thoughts, hopes and dreams. 2007 is a year that could make or break me as a person.

We were introducing the twins to Rich's children for the first time. They are the same age as Dan, Rich's eldest son.

Thursday 4 January 2007

Rich took the children back to the USA this morning, and as I drove home from the airport I experienced a feeling that was all too familiar. The same pressure and niggle under my arm, my right arm this time, as I had felt during the pre-diagnosis period under my left arm. Surely not! This could not be happening. I arranged an appointment to see someone regarding this as soon as possible. The doctor I was presented with was the wife of a member of the original medical team that I had first had the misfortune of coming across. I became fidgety, as there had been no love lost between us, and I felt I was facing the enemy once again and therefore would not be taken seriously.

Fortunately there was nothing to worry about. This, I discovered, was my first experience of cancerphobia! A condition I will suffer from for many years apparently where every tiny little tweak or pain or ache will, in my mind, be cancer. Logic will play no part in my thinking. It will just be cancer!

Friday 5 January

I received a call today from some dear friends who live overseas in Ireland and have to this point been unable to visit me but have lived every day of this nightmare with me like so many others through phone calls and emails.

'How are you doing?' they asked. 'Surviving,' I responded.

My response caught me out. Yes, I thought – I am surviving and I will survive this! It was at least a step up from my previous answers of 'existing'.

Rich returned today from the United States and I was delighted to see him – I watched him, wondering if he realised what he had taken on. Wondering why he had proposed to me – did he not realise that I may not survive and he may never get to marry me? Why was he putting himself through this? Questions I will never know the answer to – though I suspect I will one day have the nerve to ask him.

I got caught watching him and found myself struggling to explain. Did he have any idea, I wondered, how hard it is to spend time wishing that the person you adore will stop looking at you because you feel horrible, self-conscious, freak-like – and yet at the same time all you really want him to do is to look at you because he loves you? That sounds odd, I know. This is how my mind is working – confused and erratic. I must be a real pain to live with!

With the children safely back in the USA and the fun of their visit and the festivities of Christmas and our engagement over, Rich and I are forced to focus on our truly unwelcome new challenge. Life just seems so cruel sometimes. Rich and I have spent the first part of our relationship apart due to a round-the-world yacht race, and we were desperately looking forward to spending some time together as a normal couple, and then this hit us full in the face. We now begin the second year of our relationship wondering whether we will have a third.

Wednesday 10 January

Well what an odd day. I had my prosthesis fitted today – a truly odd experience. This lump of jelly, created to feel like a breast, is designed to be inserted into my bra to prevent me appearing lopsided.

I haven't gone so far as to name my prosthesis yet but 'she' and I are going to be very good friends – apparently! I presume I will become quite attached to her eventually. After all, she is a whole lot healthier than the last resident of the left side of my chest.

She is sitting in her box in our bedroom – I am not sure about her at the moment and find the whole thing too much. Stuffing something made of jelly down specially designed bras in order to make me look normal – I am not convinced yet!

She will have to wait a little.

Sunday 14 January

We joined friends of ours in London for dinner last night – six fabulous friends, three of whom I have grown up with. Jason and the twins, Lucy and James, and I go back to our very early years in Surrey. Lucy and I used to meet and roller-skate whilst our fathers played squash, and Jason and I were packed off to France each Easter to go and live with a French family in Brittany as part of an exchange, when life was simple and fun in an uncomplicated childhood. These are three people who know me very well, and in sharing my horrible circumstances with them I feel strangely safe. I am incredibly anxious, as my chemotherapy begins in a fortnight, and I still feel very vulnerable, going to great lengths to hide my lop-sided shape – and being amongst these friends is wonderful. I am drawing on all the support I can get at the moment. I am the last of the four of us to get married – Jason's wife Jo, Lucy's husband Richard and James's wife Emma have joined the team over the past three years – and we celebrated our engagement with a glass of bubbly and toasted a future we all hoped I had, although none of us said it. A positive night!

Monday 15 January

I received a picture through the post today – an image sent by Anya, Gilly's nine-year-old daughter, of what she understood to be the blowfish that was attacking her Auntie Em. I had tried to explain to her what was happening to my body without upsetting her, and her response was wonderful. It is this image that has taken hold in my mind and is now, and will continue to be, my constant enemy. It is with this picture that I shall be able to do battle. Fighting something I can see makes the whole thing just a little bit more manageable.

II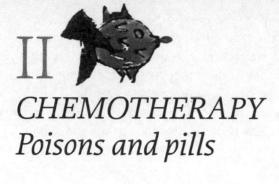

CHEMOTHERAPY
Poisons and pills

Thursday 25 January 2007

This date was firmly marked in my mind – and in my diary – for today I was due to receive the first of six doses of chemotherapy. Unprepared for what was to take place, I awoke from a very fitful sleep. I was very eager this morning to get to the hospital and get this under way. I felt that the delay I had experienced by moving the first chemotherapy appointment back at my request was wasting time. *(This change of date was due to the possibility of being able to harvest my eggs, after receiving news that I might not be able to conceive a child after chemotherapy.)*

I was eager to start the chemotherapy toxins coursing through my veins, so that they could start looking for those poisonous spines and so that I could actually feel that the medical team was doing something to chase them down and blow this thing out of the water. I feel like I have been treading water.

We arrived at the hospital and walked very slowly through the car park and in through the doors of the West Wing of Southampton General Hospital. Again no words were spoken, my little hand firmly grasped in Rich's as we wandered along the corridor to the Hamwic Ward. This was the chemotherapy day centre, and it was highly organised. On arrival we signed in and I was asked to head in to see the nurse, who took some blood and weighed me.

I was told that the reason they take blood is to ensure I am healthy enough to start chemotherapy – how ironic is that? How could I possibly be healthy, they are treating me for cancer, for heaven's sake! Anyway, it is designed to give the doctors a benchmark from which to start my treatment. My weight, again to be used as a benchmark, will allow the doctors to see how I react to the steroids that I will be receiving throughout the toxin treatment.

The morning dragged on, and eventually we were called in to see my oncologist, Dr Symonds. The results of my blood tests were back and all was well – I could begin my treatment, which, ironically, I decided was a good thing, although at no point could I ever imagine myself looking forward to chemotherapy.

I have deliberately not read any books about this treatment, frightened to face the truth again. I have ignored all the paperwork, although Rich has read it all, including all the gory details regarding the various ways in which the chemotherapy toxins could be administered – at least one of us knows what we are embarking on. I didn't want to know! Sometimes ignorance is bliss.

We returned to the waiting room and – well, waited. We waited for hours actually watching others being called through a door into the treatment area. I got impatient, fidgety and more and more terrified – it is amazing what the mind can do. Eventually there was a horrific noise – a deafening emergency siren rang out. All available staff disappeared through the treatment door, pagers bleeped, and then there was silence. A lot of frightened and panicky faces were left in the waiting room – including mine.

My oncologist called us back into his room and advised us of the situation. Behind *that* door, a patient had had an adverse reaction to a chemotherapy drug and had suffered a cardiac arrest! This did not help me one bit and I began to panic.

'Can that happen?' I asked, swallowing hard.

'Yes it can. Not everyone will experience this but there is no way of knowing who will.'

Due to this incident we were advised that my chemotherapy could not start today and could we please return tomorrow morning at 9 am. As if the build-up to this worrying stage of the treatment wasn't bad enough, this just made the whole episode worse. Once again the tears rolled down my face and I began to panic. Would this happen to me? Would I too have a cardiac arrest? Should I start chemotherapy at all? All reasoning suddenly disappeared.

Reluctantly we left and came home.

Friday 26 January

At 0400 hours this morning I sat up in bed and watched Rich leave the bedroom for a flight to Singapore and then on to Australia. A combined business trip and holiday with his children that we had planned last year, and where I was to be introduced to his family and friends – but with the diagnosis I am now sadly going to miss it all.

I held my hand out to him, tears rolling down my face, desperately wanting him to stay, reminding him that he promised he would be here for me throughout all this, that we were supposed to be fighting this together and yet he was leaving me at such a crucial point in my treatment.

As I lay in the darkness I wondered how I would ever forgive him or learn to understand that decision to leave.

A few hours later, I awoke to today's reality. It was a monumental day – I was to undergo my first dose of chemotherapy after the false start of yesterday. Loz and I left the house clutching my appointment card and some pennies for the car park. Neither one of us spoke on the journey – I felt numb and more terrified than ever after yesterday's fiasco and the terrible situation with the cardiac arrest. I had, of course, managed to convince myself overnight that it would surely happen to me! This irrationality, based mainly on the fear of the unknown, is a real nuisance and appears at every dawn.

We were the first to arrive. We were being squeezed, rather unusually, into a Friday clinic. Friday is not for breast cancer treatment but for treatment of another form of cancer. However, my oncologist was eager to get my chemotherapy under way. The room was cold and empty, and Loz and I sat waiting for further instructions.

Just as I had done yesterday I headed around the corner to be weighed and have some blood taken. I returned and sat as close to my dear friend as possible and held his hand tightly. We waited once more.

I was called to see Peter, my oncologist, who again confirmed that I was cleared to have my treatment, and we proceeded through to the treatment area – through *that* door. We had not passed through these doors yesterday and I now began to shake. Loz and I sat and waited. Tears began to roll down both our faces as we stared at each other. We were joined by a lovely chemotherapy nurse, Elaine, who was warm and gentle and caring. She could see the terror in my eyes as I explained what I had seen the day before – her patience and understanding were amazing.

Placing my right arm into a bowl of warm water so as to raise the veins in my right forearm, she sat and chatted with us about sailing in an attempt to relax me. Loz and I smiled for the first time.

With my veins behaving, Elaine explained what she was doing each and every step of the way, and with a tray of goodies sitting on her lap she began to insert a cannula into my arm and inject, incredibly slowly, a bag of bright red fluid. Unable to watch any of these steps, I locked eyes with Loz and stared at him for the next hour. Elaine slowly worked her way through three bags of fluid, one red and two clear, before hooking me up to a saline solution as a final gesture before releasing me.

As we got up to leave and head off to the oncology pharmacy to collect the various tablets and potions I would need, she advised that my first visit to the bathroom would result in bright red wee. This we found amusing, and like little children we raced off to the nearest loo in the hospital. I disappeared inside and

Loz waited, and on my return sporting a huge grin I giggled and confirmed her comments. Neither of us knew why this was funny – possibly just the release of tension.

As a treat Loz and I bought a huge sickly hot chocolate from the coffee shop near the entrance and we wandered slowly back to the car.

Back home I sat and waited. I am not sure what for exactly but I was expecting to feel something. During the evening I remember feeling a little light-headed and was anxious about this. As I slid into bed, alone, I lay there waiting. Waiting for some kind of reaction maybe to the drugs, but my mind drifted to the events of today and this evening. I measured myself, my confidence and my strength, and dozed off.

Saturday 27 January

I was not to be left alone, and so began the endless round of visiting friends and family in the guise of carers. A rota to make sure I was never on my own seemed to be in full swing. Loz was here last night obviously but left this morning, to go away, and so the next team of carers arrived in the form of my parents, on their first tour of duty. I still felt light-headed and 'floppy' – moving around the house was challenging as I grabbed hold of each wall and door, unable to let go of one until I was in contact with the next. We sat and watched the rugby and I dozed. I was still feeling horrendously light-headed and therefore very panicky. I was reminded that we had been warned that the antiemetic (sickness) drugs that they provide can cause a reaction such as mine and I began to calm a little.

Sunday 28 January

With my parents departing this morning the monitoring continued in the form of my dear friend Rach. She arrived armed with a smile and a hug. We sat and read and talked for much of today and once again I dozed – I am not sure I was much company but I was still suffering the light-headed effects of the tablets and therefore there was little I could do. Rach did not seem upset or surprised that my chitchat has reduced a little. In fact, she was probably relieved!

Monday 29 January

Rach wandered off to work this morning and I was left alone. For the past two months Team Blowfish has rallied in precision formation around me – visiting me, cooking for me, staying with me and generally attending to my every need – it has been wonderful. However, as I sit here alone now for the first time since my mastectomy in November the reality of what is happening to me is finally sinking in. I am suddenly confronted with the ugly truth of what I am dealing with and I have started to panic about the chemotherapy drugs and their reactions. Am I about to fall apart, physically, this week whilst I am alone? With both Loz and Rich away, and no carer scheduled, will I be able to handle that? It will be a crucial week for me. I guess it is going to force me to face my future without any help.

Whilst it is important to allow myself to take on board the current situation there is of course a danger in being alone. For me the danger that is prevalent in my mind is that every problem, every ache, every pain is cancer – my cancerphobia bites again. A stomach ache is clearly stomach or ovarian cancer. A neck ache, and the cancer has clearly spread up through my neck. The potential to become neurotic is huge.

As I wandered around the empty house this afternoon endeavouring to calm myself I attempted to remember the words that Peter had said as we left the hospital after our prognosis meeting at the end of November – words to the effect that every cancer patient will continue to get colds, aches and pains, just like anyone else – but that thought doesn't seem to help me because I am not 'just like anyone else' now.

Friday 2 February

I have spent today reflecting. As I look back over the past week it turns out I did not fall apart physically, I just cried a lot. For the first time I was able to let the whole thing out. I cried and cried and cried – alone with my problem, my cancer and my thoughts – the simple fact is that no matter how much help, attendance and encouragement I receive it is ultimately my disease and my challenge. It is a little like being a boxer – I have a wealth of support at every turn and a dedicated team encouraging and driving me forward, but the harsh reality is that it is me that has to go into that ring alone, and the support network has to sit, helpless, by the side of the ring and watch.

Team Blowfish consists of a cast of thousands who try to understand, and they are brilliant, but there is just one tiny little piece that even they will admit to not appreciating – and that is the abject fear I experienced when I was told the news, when I learned that people were playing with *my* life. The simple fact is that I have to sail this ship alone.

Thursday 8 February

What they don't tell you! The bastards!

The experts spend their time telling you about all the reactions you may or may not have to the poisons that they are quietly pumping into your body, but forget to tell you just how to deal with life in general whilst all this is happening. For example, they tell that you may feel sick without the antiemetic tablets but forget to mention that they will make you feel so light-headed you will not be able to move. They forget to mention that you may not feel like eating for the first two days after each dose of chemo, but conscious that eating is a good thing you try to do so – but they don't mention that if you do eat you will experience indigestion that makes you cry with every mouthful and every drop of water you swallow – these as a result of the delightful steroids they advise you take to stop yourself feeling sick!

They advise you that you may feel achy as with a heavy dose of flu but they don't mention the crippling stomach cramps that are a combination of the steroids and the sheer level of fear you experience.

Your skin will react in a fashion you never saw as a teenager, your emotions are in turmoil and you become irrational and unbearable and incredibly frustrated.

In short, they don't tell you how to face the world, how to look at yourself in the mirror, or how to face the man you adore – hoping he will still love you.

These are the facts that I need!

Whilst I appreciate that every patient is different, surely they could give us all a heads-up.

Saturday 10 February

Shock and pain – individually they are designed to paralyse, but as a double act the results are truly stunning! Together, they wipe you out at the knees with maximum effect – a truly unpleasant combination – and today I experienced their full force.

This disease is many things, not least cruel. You expend all your efforts telling yourself that you are okay, that you look alright when you know you don't, that you can do this when you think you can't, that life will resume as normal and that you must be strong, brave and push on through. You strive to continue and learn to deal with new situations, and then wallop – another heavy step through this long line of shit – hair loss!

Don't get me wrong – this is not a surprise, I knew it was coming. I had arranged to meet my friend Jenny in London this morning, and together we visited my hairdresser to face another brutal stage of this cancer. I was to have my head shaved.

I had taken a shower this morning and as usual I washed my hair. This turned out to be a terrible idea as it was today, of all days, that my hair decided to fall out. The shampoo would not wash out and my hair matted itself into knotted chunks. In desperation I stood under the running shower running my hands over the mess on my head. Trying desperately to untangle the knots, I took a comb and tried to brush them out, tears streaming down my face as the reality of my cancer took hold – again. The panic rushed through me – my hair was falling out and there was nothing I could do about it.

I stumbled out of the shower and sat motionless on the loo seat feeling dizzy and spaced out – I was alone in the house and I needed help. I was terrified.

After a very tearful drive up to London I caught up with Jenny. Our first stop of the day was a large department store. We were wig shopping.

There is something very different about dress-up and reality. As a child I used to love dressing up and escaping into another world in my imagination with different clothes, make-up, shoes and wigs – but now, suddenly faced with the fact that this wig was not part of dressing up but a tangible part of my illness, I could not face the truth. I cried and cried whilst the poor shop assistant placed wig after wig on my balding head – the hair still in knotted chunks from the shower this morning.

We spent the rest of the day shopping, nipping in and out of various stores looking for nothing in particular, and at the end of the day together we headed for the hairdressers.

It was the end of a very busy Saturday as we arrived to an empty salon and were met by Sheramin, long-standing hairdresser and friend. She took us into a back room and with very little discussion, as there was nothing to say, she took her clippers and began to shave my hair, the hair she has, for fifteen years, rescued from various hair disasters and lovingly cut and shaped into such wonderful styles.

I held Jenny's hand so tightly and squeezed so hard I was sure

I was draining the blood from her hand and breaking her fingers for that matter too. As my nails sank deeper into the now red raw flesh of her hand, my head lowered in shame, tears rolled down my face as I watched my beautiful blonde bob falling in chunks at my feet. It was soul-destroying. I have lost my boob, which is devastating enough – a part of me that makes me feel feminine – and now the hair too. It was only a matter of time before the eyelashes fell out. This cancer was, slowly but steadily, breaking me.

After removing my hair Sheramin turned to my wig. Unwilling to face the reality of a wig, I fought her requests as I don't like it – it is blonde but it is long and is not me – but then I doubt if I would be happy with any wig at this point. However, the girls convinced me that I should put it on, and I agreed that Sheramin should cut the wig into my hair style. She cut and shaped the wig into the bob she had just shaved – it was much better – but I still vowed I would never wear it!

I lay in bed in the dark thinking about the events of today. I did wear the wig for a few hours at my evening appointment, but I felt ridiculous and more determined than ever not to wear it again.

Hair loss is quite definitely the most fundamentally challenging part of this nightmare so far. Perhaps surprisingly, it is not the loss of the left breast but my hair that makes me feel so freakish. I am able to conceal my butchered form behind layers of clothing, but it is so much harder to hide the baldness.

I am sure I will get used to this, but today was horrific.

Before closing my eyes, I concluded that this disease moves very quickly to your head. It gets inside your mind and takes hold of your thoughts, controlling all things rational – the ability to think like an adult, a gift I have had for many years, disappears! Cancer gets inside and destroys you. All logical progressive and positive thoughts vanish.

Sunday 11 February

Two friends of mine, Rach and Billy, moved into a new house this weekend just along the beach front from us. They had suggested I pop round for a wee glass of bubbly. This terrified me! Go outside! Without hair! Alone and with no support! NEVER! I could not do that and was not ready. I stalled and stalled, using any reason to not leave the house – I fiddled around moving things from place to place, putting stuff away that should have been put away months ago. It was in fact an extremely efficient hour, but after a second call I told them my problem.

They told me that I would be amongst friends so it would all be okay. So I left the house, drove around to see their lovely new home and sat in the car for about fifteen minutes. So nearly there!

Finally inside, we raised a glass – and then came the advice. I admit that I am new to this bandana business and clearly, according to my very trendy friend Billy, I was not wearing it properly. After much fiddling around with it he suggested that my ears should not be tucked into the bandana and should be removed outside. This was a very bad move. Through the tears of laughter, which lasted some considerable time I might add, instructions to reinstall the ears inside the bandana came as I apparently took on the look of Yoda! Picture that if you can. Not a good look for anyone, I must say. It was decided that a new bandana should be purchased, and as I left I promised to do so.

I had a very teary conversation with Rich this evening before bed. He is still in Australia and I miss him terribly. This weekend has been shattering – losing my hair has really knocked me and my confidence, it is heart-wrenching. There were no words from Rich that could make this any easier, but to be told that the man you adore loves you with or without hair in the same way that he loves you with or without a boob does help a little.

Monday 12 February

My light was shining. My day had dawned. And I was so excited I could barely breathe. This is what I had been focusing on and waiting for. The frustrations of sitting at home, watching others go to work, hearing their stories of a shit day in the office were over – it was my turn again!

I thought hard about the commitment that both Simon and Tim had made to me, and thought it was remarkable. Simon had a choice back in November to leave me to recover and select a new training mate who was in an easier less complicated situation, or to honour their commitment of employment to me. I was delighted that they decided to behave in an honourable fashion. Apparently it was never an option for them to renege on their offer of last year – but I still held my breath each time the office called during my time off the water, a little part of me still expecting the worst, and I think I would actually have understood it if they had called to retract their offer. After all, they needed commitment from their training skippers and mates, a commitment I was unable to give as I did not know how my body would react to chemotherapy.

After all, I had two options on offer to me with this chemotherapy – Option A: Swing the lead, or Option B: Bust an arse. Me? Option B, and they knew it! They knew me, they knew I could do the job, and they knew what made me tick. They had watched me go down in this horrific nightmare and were watching me come back up again and they stuck by me – I was delighted.

I challenge anyone to resent me the smile I wear today.

I spent the day thanking them – anyone and everyone that I saw actually – for honouring that commitment. It didn't matter who they were, I was just pleased to be back.

My first day on the water, however, would be Monday 26 February. I have to wait two more painfully frustrating weeks before I can slip those lines, and I am incredibly impatient. I will have had my second dose of chemotherapy by then, which makes me fidgety and impatient, and now nauseous too. Brilliant!

Wednesday 14 February

Valentine's Day! Loz and I decided that, in the absence of his girlfriend and my fiancé, we would go out for dinner together. We booked a table in a restaurant in Hamble and in an attempt to dress up and look smart I abandoned my now familiar pink bandana and sported a delightful pale blue pashmina number coiled up and knotted on my head – it was an interesting look that an African woman of the plains would have been proud of – but at least the colour matched my belt buckle! Loz didn't snigger once. Bless him!

After a wonderful evening talking about everything but cancer we sauntered across the cobbled street and into the pub to join some of our other friends – many of whom had not seen me since the diagnosis and whose faces spoke volumes.

Thursday 15 February

Chemo Thursday had arrived. Dose Number Two, and with Rich still away Mummy and Loz were on call. So together, armed with the obligatory chemotherapy appointment card, tablets, car parking and hot chocolate money, we headed off to Southampton General Hospital once more.

It was back to the now familiar Hamwic Ward, but today was different. Today was the first time I had been to the clinic with no hair and I now looked like everyone else. I felt very self-conscious as familiar faces smiled at me but I didn't smile back. I do not want to be a part of this group – a member of the breast cancer group.

I was sent off to be weighed and to have my bloods taken to see if my white blood cell count was good and to check that I was not suffering from neutropenia – a condition that affects the body's ability to fight infection. If the blood count had been low then I would not have been able to have my chemotherapy today and would have to wait another week for the neutrophils to increase.

However, all was good today. My weight hadn't changed at all – still 62 kilos – and no neutropenia in sight.

Today was my mother's first experience of the chemotherapy, and I was glad she was here. I want to bring both my parents, individually, so that they can be involved and try to understand what their daughter is going through. I was a little calmer than last time – not much though. Loz and Mummy spent the day trying to keep my mind off the episode. I had a particularly unfriendly nurse today who was more interested in leaving in time to collect her children than administering my poisons gently and carefully, and after knocking my cannula needle, causing me extreme pain, and showing a level of frustration and a complete lack of understanding as to why I was crying she was replaced, fortunately, by my first week's angel, who was gentle and sympathetic to the core.

When one is attached to machinery and therefore restricted in one's movement there is little one can do – but had I been able to move she would have moved faster!

———

Two down, four to go! Mmm – that doesn't sound very progressive, does it? Well to me at times it is massive, and then I remember just how long I have been living with this and I go into despair. We are only in February, and I have until the end of June – four months to go!

I mentioned my light-headedness to Peter this morning, and I was advised that these particular tablets should not be given to patients under the age of fifty! I was speechless, but with a change of tablet I crossed my fingers that I would not feel so 'floppy'.

We also learnt something new today – almost free car parking! Our last visit had cost me around £8.00 for the day to park and be put through the chemotherapy day-centre mill. However, this week we have been told that we can have our ticket stamped and the whole episode need only cost £1.00. Wouldn't it have been nice if someone had mentioned this to us?

Friday 16 February

I noticed my loss of hair tremendously today. I am a hair curler. Since I was a child I have twisted my hair. I used to suck my right thumb and twist and curl my hair with the left one. It was something I did when I was tired and it was a comforter too – and never have I needed more comforting than now. I am in desperate need of some hair curling. At thirty-six years old you would think I might have grown out of this, but no! Don't laugh, when I was tiny I curled my hair into such a knot I had to have my finger cut out as my parents couldn't undo the mess their little daughter had managed to create. Standing crying in my cot with my finger stuck to the side of my head – I must have been a picture! How I would love to be curling my hair right now! I have ditched the thumb sucking, though.

Saturday 17 February

Today I have developed what I lovingly refer to as 'the wobbles'. These are moments when I feel I cannot cope. I tend to burst into tears for no reason. My wobbles can last for anything from five minutes to five hours. They just take hold of me – when I am least expecting it – and I simply have no control.

The solution to these wobbles is not known yet. Sadly, a hug can result in making the whole thing worse. Sensitivity is not always the best policy, and the truth is often better. My brother is my solution to everything. When I am finding the whole episode too much and too overwhelming to deal with I just telephone Rupert. He is always on the other end of the line – he continues with his promise of calling me religiously every night and every morning from wherever he is, without a thought to his situation or location or the demands on his time as a working husband and father of six-year-old twins.

This morning I was struggling and was not handling being alone. With Rich away and my demands on Loz relentless I am trying not to bother him too much, so in an attempt to share the burden of me I called Rupes – again! I worry about Loz straining under the tugs of emotions. After all, he has a life, and I am a part of it, but my demands on his time are becoming all-consuming as my wobbles are becoming more and more frequent. It must be very hard living with me at the moment.

Between them, the boys have worked admirably throughout this quagmire of cancer during these early stages – but I think both will be pleased when Rich returns.

After a brief chat with my folks this morning too I decided to drive up to see them. A dose of tender loving care from them was just what I needed. It was the first time that they had seen me with my bandana on but I refused to show them my bald head – the last time I was bald I was about two months old and it was these two wonderful people who saw me that way then, and yet I was not brave enough to show them today – not yet at least.

I am delighted to say that my parents have now moved out of my brother's caravan and back into the house, which now has four walls and a roof, at least, but remains a work in progress.

Daddy and I went for a short walk around the village. It is just two days since my second dose of chemotherapy, and it is for these following three days that I have a tendency to feel light-headed, but I have worked out that as long as I have my bananas then I seem to be alright. So, with me clutching my banana and holding my father's arm so tightly, we wandered very gently down the drive and through the village for a leg stretch. It was a lovely tender moment between father and daughter where words were absent and the love just took over. He never let go of my arm – not once. We bumped into a friend and popped in for coffee, or a glass of water in my case – another craving resulting from the chemo toxins – give me a banana and some water and I am a happy girl!

It is three in the morning as I write this and I am awake – wide awake! I removed my bandana once the bedside light was out and fell asleep. After a few hours I have woken up needing to use the bathroom. The room is lit by the moonlight and therefore I did not turn on any lights but wandered off to the *en suite*. On my return I saw a bald-headed image in the doorway. I assume it is my father, who must have heard me get up, and I began to talk to him. After a short moment I realise that it is my own reflection in the mirror over the basin and I am, in fact, alone. It was a horrible moment of reality and fear. Now I cannot sleep.

Saturday 24 February

I felt like a freak show today. I was out and about in my bandana, and it is clear, beyond question, that there is something wrong with me. People can tell that I have no hair and that I am not just sporting my bandana as a fashion statement, and yet it sparks their imagination, interest and excitement. They stare and stare and I have nowhere to hide. That is the sad truth about how humans work. They stare at the unusual, and I look unusual.

Monday 26 February

Brilliant! Today had finally arrived. My first day on the water since this cancer nightmare began. I was assigned to a skipper whom I knew very well, which was wonderful.

We were sent out to play in the Solent. Our team on board was a group of people who have signed up to sail part or all of a round-the-world yacht race, and it was our job to train them in the rudiments (black art) of sail trim and wind awareness, along with a basic grounding in safety and navigation, before they set sail on their epic journey. For many this was their first experience of sailing, which would be a huge challenge and very exciting on a large yacht.

I had a ball out there. It blew its tits off – or technically speaking, from my point of view, it blew its tit off – but I didn't care. It was bloody fantastic! And just as I thought, it made me feel alive, like the cancer had never happened. Like this whole episode was just a bad dream of horrific proportions. I handle this disease in my head by taking small achievable steps. 12 February was one of those all-important steps, and today was another. I know that now, but on that miserable cold, dark painful day in November it was all I could do to keep focused.

Today on the water was absolutely amazing – it was the difference between being alive and feeling alive.

Monday 5 March

We had a wonderful week putting the trainee sailors through their paces with day sailing and evening lectures. I found myself grinning almost all week, with the exception of the odd wobble and a dose of sheer exhaustion during the first evening lecture last Tuesday. Fortunately the skipper, Danny, was a star and together we battled my cancer and my reactions to it and I was delighted. I returned home this afternoon feeling very successful.

Thursday 8 March

Third dose of chemo today, and Rich's first real visit to the weed-killer clinic – his first visit through *those* doors. He was a familiar sight for Peter, and after once again confirming that I was not neutropenic we were off to pastures new. I didn't cry much this time but I was reminded that this was my final dose of the combination of drugs that I have been on, and that it will change next visit. There will be new drugs and therefore new fears.

They don't mention that the steroids will up the ante on your hunger somewhat. As responsible adults they really should point out that you will do a weekly shop that will put shame to the masses and would in fact feed a small African nation.

With Rich home I noticed something today and laughed – I never believed the day would come when I would eat as much as he! As I settled down for my umpteenth meal of the day, I pottered about the house writing and preparing for my next week on the water. My desire for food has not diminished as time moves on – I continue to send down for bananas and other tasty treats in the middle of the night.

Rich asked when lunch would be. I suggested noon but I advised that I would have eaten at least three times before that should he wish to join me. Basically, should he pop his head into the kitchen at any point during the morning there would be food available at any time.

Bless him though, he is putting up a true and good fight, matching banana for banana with his ravenous fiancée. However, if there is a plus side to wiping the supermarket shelves clean of bananas, cheese biscuits, tomatoes, red grapes (and the odd jelly baby), it is that I haven't put on any weight – my metabolism perhaps? However, I doubt if I would pass a drugs test on banned substances and steroids for the next Olympic eating team.

Wind! A factor that the medicos forget to mention and really should for the sake of all around you. Chemotherapy is to blame apparently. It is the excuse for everything. Me – a girl who clearly does not partake in that type of windy activity – and before you all get on your soap boxes shouting from the rafters that I do – I don't! Because, quite simply, I am a girl and as we all know girls smell of roses so they cannot!

Saturday 10 March

I waited patiently, and excitedly, for the familiar feelings that I know come after a dose of chemotherapy. The symptoms that confirm that the chemo drugs are doing their thing, the tingling in my gums, the gentle change in taste, the heartburn, the burning tongue caused by the mint in my toothpaste. These symptoms all take place over a period of about seven days and all help me to believe that the drugs are working – seeking out the poisonous blowfish spines and zapping them.

This may seem like a childish image but it works for me.

Staring at myself in the mirror I release a huge sigh. I cannot wait to reclaim what this blowfish thought it could steal from me!

Sunday 18 March

Apparently bald is beautiful. You have all read the papers this morning and will have noted the new hair image of the young singing celebrity sensation that is Britney Spears. Her baldness comes just a couple of weeks after my head-shaving episode and I am therefore clearly ahead of my time – a trend setter and obviously a huuuuge influence on the rich and famous!

However, despite that, and in a desperate attempt to help me look a little less like a refugee or a woman of the hills (minus floral dress and basket) and more like an international ever-so-slightly-sexy yachtswoman, I need help!

I challenged my friends and family today. I am in desperate need of some ideas. The bandana look is fine for certain functions, and life back on the water in chilly spring means that everyone is wearing a hat so I feel a little less conspicuous out there – but any thoughts about off-the-water headwear would be gratefully received.

I was told recently by a dear friend of mine that I am more

than just blonde hair, boobs and legs – which is handy really as I only appear to have one of those three left at the moment. Nevertheless I would dearly love to be able to feel just a teeny bit feminine every now and again!

I have another three months before I can take on the Kylie look of very short CURLY hair.

Thursday 29 March

Dose Number Four and I felt pathetic. There I was reclining on the now familiar and rather unpleasant blue plastic chair, rigid with fear today as there was a drug change! You see, you become comfortable with the familiar, and for me my FEC combination was familiar – I knew how I reacted, I knew what it felt like going in and I understood the recovery period for the following days – but a change in drug brought a change in circumstances. This was the drug that was being administered to that poor lady on the horrible day in January when I went for my first chemotherapy appointment who then suffered a cardiac arrest – the memory of which will never fade for me. So, imagining the worst, I sat shaking as they hooked me up to the new dose of poisons that was supposed to make me better – wallowing in a small amount of self-pity and massive dose of fear for the potential reaction – I prepared myself for a horrific response and began the usual clock watching and waited.

I was advised that I should relax, and that if I was going to have a reaction I was in the best place for this to happen. That didn't help me one bit.

I was also advised that the poison that goes into this new drug is derived from the yew tree – a poisonous tree found in most churchyards.

As the hour ticked by I noticed that I had no reaction, nothing! So we left the hospital this afternoon comfortable in the knowledge that in the future I would be able to go into any churchyard and lick any yew tree I fancy. Fabulous!

During today's visit Rich and I spoke with a woman in the next-door chair – her story was so much worse than mine and made me feel like a child, like I should grow up and get a grip. Each of my scheduled doses of toxins takes one hour to administer and there are only six over a period of four months. The woman I spoke to today had been diagnosed with a second type of cancer following her original breast cancer diagnosis and was therefore undergoing her second round of chemotherapy, which lasts a whole year with each dose taking seven hours to administer. It is people like her who make me feel pathetic.

Rich and I looked at one another, listening in horror to this poor woman pouring out her feelings, and our faces spoke volumes – stop moaning!

Monday 2 April

Today I felt like a failure. I had let the cancer, the chemotherapy and the symptoms attached to it take control. Or so I thought.

Every joint in my body ached today, the stomach cramps that took control of me towards the end of yesterday evening had not let up, and sleep eluded me, providing a night of turmoil. Reluctantly I succumbed to Rich's suggestion of doing nothing today and, feeling like a failure, I shuffled downstairs in my jammies to embark on a day curled up in a ball on the sofa. I found this was the only way to reduce the spasms that were part and parcel of this delightful new chapter in my treatment with the new drug.

It was a very frustrating time. Rich was upstairs working and I reluctantly had to call for his attention. As I was unable to move from my ball-like position on the sofa he dug out the 'Beating the Blowfish' file stored discreetly on the bookcase in the sitting room. Amongst all the papers that were stuffed into my hot little mitts when this nightmare began was a note which contained a number – the hotline number to my relief and support and encouragement from the experts, and it was this piece of paper that we sought now. An eleven-digit number, my emergency line, and a number that I foolishly believed would help – a last resort, but what a mistake!

Careful to acknowledge that all the symptoms and reactions that I was feeling can be developed by anyone, whether suffering from cancer or not – indigestion, mouth ulcers, sore joints, period pains etc. I also remembered that through my chemotherapy these symptoms have been magnified, resulting in the need for extra-strong special medication to counteract the symptoms. A trip to a local doctor and the release of a regular prescription drug does not solve the problem – so you will therefore be surprised to learn that when, in my state of crippled sofa-hugging spasms, I telephoned the magic hotline number for advice on my state and drug options for this particular little concern of mine I was told to pop down to my local surgery and have a blood test. Brilliant!

I personally found this frustrating and disappointing. This response from the experts saddened me and I lost just a little tiny bit of faith in them. I had been told by my oncologist on Thursday, at the first administration of my new drug, that symptoms such as this could exist, and their inability to address my situation was irritating.

I checked myself in the mirror before undressing this evening, and I concluded that I now do look like the refugee I have spoken of. I felt like a ninety-year-old lady too. Let's hope I make it to that age.

Tuesday 3 April

Who was it that said chemo was treating me well? Oh yes, it was me. Well I lied! It is rubbish! After all the horror stories I have heard I realise I have been very lucky to date and I guess it is my turn now.

I sadly have to admit that my fears have been confirmed – this cancer shit did bite me in the arse after all, and in spectacular fashion.

Each day is understandably a new challenge, and this new drug presented just that today – and the discovery of a pain threshold I never realised I had. I also revisited the well-known concept that too much sofa time results in too much thinking time, and that is pretty much all I did today. My thoughts turned to our wedding. Dare I think about such a beautiful day I was not sure I would ever reach? Sometimes I feel like I will and sometimes, when every now and then I catch myself in the mirror, I lose my confidence and start with the questions once more. Why did he propose? Is it because I am sick? I know he loves me, but does he pity me? Is our wedding day his gift to me before it is all too late? A special day every girl wants – the chance to feel like a princess. Oh my God the same damn questions. I know all the answers but I still ask myself.

With those thoughts still burning in my mind I steeled myself to look through the mountain of wedding magazines that have gathered in little corners around the house. I have previously been too afraid to open them and peek inside at a world I am afraid I will not get the chance to be involved in – not daring to think of 12 July 2008, just in case.

It was a very tough but rewarding step for me – I actually gained a little more determination to reach my wedding day.

Excitedly I called Gilly this afternoon. Despite her continuous protestations of letting me down and her frustrations about being absent throughout my treatment, she is, I believe, finally beginning to realise that despite living over two hundred miles north of me she is vital to my recovery, and the constant phone calls are support enough.

She is a woman with the world on her plate right now with her own family challenges, three wonderful but enormously active and demanding children, a job, a husband, a house to run and a social life that puts mine to shame. However, despite all that this wonderful woman has found time to provide me with a dose of reality and grounding in this crazy situation I find myself in. She is great for me and I miss her.

I called her because I wanted to talk about my wedding – finally!

As I popped pill after pill, whimpering on the sofa, waiting for something to happen, for the pain to reduce, my tear-stained face buried once more in another cushion, I wondered how people ever manage without painkillers, the attention of a good man and the support of great friends. I could not do this alone. After a few more minutes of self-pity I got a grip and settled into another terrible murder mystery challenge for Dick van Dyke in *Diagnosis Murder*. You see – sofa time is very bad for me!

As I lie here in bed, writing my thoughts, which continue to range from the sublime to the ridiculous, I feel frustrated, fractious and exhausted. They say everything happens for a reason. Has this episode reduced my risk of heart attack or a stroke? Has it lowered my cholesterol level, or reduced my chance of developing lung cancer because it has made me address my body, which is a phenomenal machine I have always been afraid of? It has certainly encouraged me to address any little issues. Perhaps this adventure has saved my life?

These are questions I will never know the answers to, and really I have stopped asking them, but I note them down just the same. I have been reading today about my new drug – docetaxel – and I am trying to understand exactly what is going on. Why have they altered the course of drugs? Is it simply to challenge any remaining cancerous cells as they become complacent and resistant to the FEC combination? Note to self: ask Peter.

Wednesday 11 April

It is amazing how fellow chemo patients can spot another chemo patient at ten paces. I was today accosted by a woman in Marks & Spencer who asked me how long I had being having chemotherapy, when my mastectomy took place – and then she proceeded to show me her left boob, or rather the site where her left boob had been before her own mastectomy. She had a scar which she was very proud of!

Unwilling to offend, I glanced down to inspect. I did not spend too much time as I am still finding it very difficult to look at my chest and scar and am definitely still struggling with my own lopsidedness, let alone that of a stranger. *Plus* I am not one for checking out the chest walls of complete strangers in a crowded store – or anywhere else for that matter. I have moved on from my obsession with staring longingly at the cleavages of strange women I have never met before.

Thursday 19 April

Any parent reading this will understand these words. I, however, do not completely. I am not a parent, and in this situation I am most definitely the child.

Today I took my father to my penultimate dose of chemotherapy – a deliberate act on my part but one that I knew would challenge both of us. I am not sure I will ever know if it was the right thing to do but I wanted both my parents to be a part of this chemotherapy and understand what I have been through. My father will admit that he is not good with all things medical, and whilst I was not aiming to frighten him I did want him to be a part of all of this, to understand me.

A dose of chemotherapy is shocking to watch helplessly from the sidelines for anyone, but for a parent it must be very hard. We talked all the time and I took up my usual stance of not looking at the nurse but locked eyes with Daddy. After a painful hour we left, via the oncology pharmacy, and breathed a sigh of relief.

One more dose to go.

Friday 20 April

Throughout all this chemotherapy stuff with the nurses systematically poisoning my system I note that I have developed a craving for certain foods immediately after each dose: bananas, tomatoes, mint imperials. Well today I noted that I appear to have gone through the need to have certain types of food but I must admit I have completely fallen in love with natural yoghurt. Don't laugh. I have developed a deep love for it and it works for me so I am clinging on and sitting tight.

Tuesday 24 April

I spent today in London. I had a meeting with a friend at noon and arrived early.

I got off the Southampton train at Waterloo and was plunged into familiar chaos – I stood still for some minutes with people rushing around, pushing me from one side of the platform to the other as they charged past and disappeared down below to the Underground. The chaos triggered a memory, a memory that I struggled to place initially. It was like a scene from a movie I had once seen, and then it hit me – this is how my life used to be, the rushing and charging around, the urgency to be somewhere else as quickly as possible. I used to travel on the Underground twice a day – to and from my city office, walking with an immense sense of urgency, my head buried in a book, even as I walked – a book that would take me miles from this place. Today was like looking in through a window.

I took a Tube to Bond Street and found myself smiling. I used to know the Underground backwards, the various lines and all their little tricks. Hell I used to know exactly where to stand on a platform in order to be in front of a door, and, more alarmingly, I used to care!

I alighted and, in the heat of the day, I ambled slowly down Oxford Street, fidgeting in my heels and smart woollen suit with my black woollen pashmina on my head. I wandered in and out of shops browsing. I hate shopping but I was killing time. It wasn't long before I gave up, though, as I was hot and uncomfortable, so I disappeared into one store and, without trying anything on, purchased a pair of jeans, a polo shirt and a pair of black flip-flops. These I would save until later, after the meeting.

It was a glorious day and I sat, hideously overdressed, in black trousers and a woollen cream jacket – plus mac. I was blowing my nose continuously and was rapidly loosing my taste. I sat staring through streaming eyes hidden behind dark Jackie Onassis sunglasses surreptitiously watching the workforce of the city escaping the drudgery of their offices for one tiny minute, variously chatting, reading and generally enjoying the outside. I saw me, ten years earlier.

I was watching life go by rather than taking part in it – and for all my health issues at the moment I would never have traded my position with theirs. It simply reaffirmed my decision to leave.

I met with my friend and we wandered together to the meeting venue, chatting.

After the meeting, everyone left and I sat and finished my tea and then waited. At the earliest opportunity I shot into the large toilet in Starbucks and changed into the jeans, polo shirt and flip-flops I had earlier bought – and immediately felt my blood pressure drop. I felt comfortable and relaxed. Now don't get me wrong, I can look great in a suit – but only when I have to!

Please don't misunderstand me. I did enjoy my time in the City but my tolerance of it runs out very quickly these days. I think I suffer from claustrophobia and the Underground made me feel suffocated as it disappeared lower and lower beneath the pavements.

As I sat in the 'Drain' – the branch of the Underground that travels directly from Waterloo to the financial heart of the City and which was part of my regular daily route from my home in Battersea to my desk in Broadgate – wearing flip-flops and jeans I was doing the one thing that I used to be terrified of, and that was standing out.

I had at last put my head above the parapet, and I felt liberated. I had come full circle.

Wednesday 25 April

It is all about the numbers. I sat outside our local pub tonight with my dear friend Gail, eyes wide open, whilst she patiently counted the number of eyelashes I had left to paint blue with mascara in a vain but desperate attempt to make me look like a girl rather than a freak.

The results are:

	Left	Right
Top	27	32
Bottom	13	16

I thought about some more numbers when I got home. These figures represent my diagnosis and treatment so far:

1	Number of chemo doses left
2	Number of weeks to my dose
6	Number of months since the bottom fell out of my world
15	Number of radiotherapy doses to come
72	Number of days to the start of radiotherapy
Endless	Number of times I have asked myself why me?

I considered the first in that line of numbers, and with renewed vigour I turned out the light.

Thursday 26 April

Today I noted my confidence levels. My confidence is dwindling. I note that as my eyelashes slowly but unfailingly fall out one by one I become more and more embarrassed by my appearance, spending much of my time looking down avoiding the looks of whomever I am talking to. I note too that I will do anything not to look at someone, content in the memory of the childlike belief that if I do not look at someone they will not be able to see me. This is ironic really, as a dear friend has commented to me that my baldness makes my eyes stand out.

Fortunately, the sunglasses that I wear daily for my job prove to be a godsend. I do not look odd wearing glasses all day, as all sailors where sunglasses. It also helps because the combination of wind and chemotherapy drugs results in unbearably watery eyes, which is proving to be my worst symptom so far.

I find myself relying more and more on the anonymity gained from hiding behind my sunglasses.

Tuesday 1 May

Once again I am back on the water battling the elements of the infamous Solent – the waves thrashing against the boat, water hurtling down the deck devastating all in its path ... No, seriously, I am back out on the water today but the Solent is not misbehaving. In fact there is absolutely no wind at all! I am training another group of novice crew who have decided to take on the rigours of crossing an ocean, in preparation for their upcoming race. It is my job to train these souls to handle the elements, and that training begins here in Southampton. Sadly, however, this whole week is forecast to be still, calm, warm and sunny. Great for the suntan but not so great for training a sailing team.

It is my birthday this week. I am glad I have made it to thirty-seven years old, and I am glad that I will be spending it sailing.

Friday 4 May

After the challenge that I issued previously to my friends and family regarding headwear I have been sent an array of items that have been quite interesting. However, the best was given to me today.

Today is my birthday, and I have been out on the water once again training the new recruits. There have been four boats out training with us. As a fleet we all berthed in the same marina, and after eating our dinner on board our yachts this evening we gathered en masse in a local pub to celebrate. I was joined by Rich, who was berthed in the same marina, and it was at this point that I was handed possibly the most ridiculous headwear item I have seen – but the most lovingly made. During dinner a dear friend, Hannah, who was the skipper of one of the other yachts, had decided to make a headpiece for me – to include new hair! It was a truly Heath Robinson affair with lengths of string that had been attached to a j-cloth. The string had been plaited and had a bow at the end of each plait. The charming blue and white cloth had been tacked loosely into a shape that vaguely, just, resembled a circle so that it could sit proudly on my head. Attached to the front of the j-cloth was a piece of paper with my name on it, so it was personalised too!

Thursday 10 May

Today was an extraordinary day for many reasons, not least as we pushed forward through Phase Two of this cancer nightmare – the chemotherapy – and checked out of the clinic for what will hopefully be the last time.

For one final time, I ambled down the long corridor from the entrance on Floor B to the Hamwic Ward. For one final time I gave blood, clearly reluctantly as it turns out as it took the efforts of four nurses before a cannula could finally be inserted into the tired, hard, overworked and unreceptive veins of my right arm. For one final time I visited my oncologist, Peter, to hear the news that I could have my final dose of poisons as planned. I prayed that I wasn't neutropenic.

Rich and I entered the sterile treatment room and once again we sat and waited. Another woman followed us in shortly after and sat down beside me. Quite frankly she looked terrible. She looked drawn and tired, thin and desperate. Her posture said it all. There was a distinct lack of sparkle. She had a boy of around nine with her – her son I presumed – who sat with her, fidgeting, and began to read to her.

For some weeks now I have been trying to understand what people have meant when they have said that I look great, that I still have my sparkle and that I do not look ill at all. I have not been able to understand their words as I believe that I look exactly like any cancer patient undergoing chemotherapy. Well it suddenly all became clear to me when I looked across at this poor woman. In fact I did not look like a cancer patient but a trendy young thing who chooses to wear a bandana. It is moments like this that are pure heaven to someone like me and must be cherished. I smiled.

When the same wonderfully kind Elaine wandered over to us clutching her tray of goodies I decided that it was going to be a great day. She said she would be looking after me for my last appointment, which was just perfect. She was always gentle and held my confidence.

I have had no idea really what goes on underneath the pillow she has put over her hands since the first dose to shield me from what she is doing. I have always chosen to remain in my own little world with my head down and facing away from the reality of what is taking place through the tubes in my right arm. We always spoke continuously but I never looked. I would stare desperately at my companion – my father, my mother, Rich or Loz – anything to avoid the reality. Well not today. Today I finally managed to steel myself to lift my head to look at my nurse, and to look around the room too on this significant date – a place I had visited on five previous occasions and a place I hated and couldn't wait to see the back of.

One hour later it was all over. I had officially checked out of the weedkiller clinic. As I left the hospital, wrapped in the warmth and safety of Rich's arms, with tears of relief streaming down my face I turned and looked back over my right shoulder. I looked back towards a room I hoped never to see again, a room that I shall, however, miss just a tiny bit for its drive and focus on living and life itself.

Whilst I did not enjoy my regular visits to the Hamwic Ward, for obvious reasons, with its needles and its poisons, I shall miss it just a little bit too. I did – unintentionally and unwillingly – find a familiarity about the place that I hoped never to become comfortable with, and as I left today memories flooded my mind of my time there – trapped in that ghastly waiting room, clutching my dog-eared appointment card, surrounded by women – some cheery, others wrapped in cuddles from their loved ones, hiding faces containing the devastating news that I hoped never to receive. I remember the wait, the eternal wait, for the call for the weigh-in, the blood test and then finally the consultation with my oncologist who would give that all important nod for the day's dose of chemotherapy toxins. And finally, I remember the call of my name, the invitation to go through to the sterile environment of the treatment room with rows of patients hooked up to their drips and lines, some sleeping, some chatting but all wearing faces of anxiety. Today that all ended and I was glad.

I think it was the people within that clinic who have helped me smile through the tears over the last six months. They have helped me face the task and handle the enormity of my challenge.

Still, we said our fond goodbyes this afternoon. I don't think I ever thought that I would make today. It seemed such a long way off. I certainly couldn't see it before. I am another year older and a lifetime wiser and healthier. I hadn't envisaged being bald at any point in my life either. Hell, I hadn't envisaged spending any of my life with just one boob – I mean, they come in pairs, don't they? Some things just do – legs, arms, boobs – but here I am checking out of the chemotherapy clinic – bald and boobless!

Plonked on the sofa back at the ranch later I reflected on today. It has been a highly emotional one for both Rich and me but a huge step in the right direction. Onwards to fun-filled days of hair washing, mascara wearing and taking on the general look of a female once more. Oh, and there is the small matter of fifteen doses of radiotherapy too.

Another day, another challenge.

I noted today that Rich had spent some time writing beside me in a pink notepad that I carried around. It was not until tonight that I looked at the words he had written. They read:

'Rich was very busy today but fortunately he is lovely and tolerated my behaviour, beautifully as always.'

All I have to say is, 'Cheeky monkey!'

Friday 11 May

Yesterday I went to what I hope will be my final chemotherapy appointment. I have since been thinking a great deal and want to acknowledge the nursing staff who have helped me through this – their guidance, encouragement, tolerance and support in getting me this far have been faultless – it is impossible to put into words my feelings really except to say that I am here because of them.

It is amazing what you can enjoy in this world. This morning I filed my chemotherapy appointment card in the file at home, which for me was an enormous landmark and one that just made me smile so much.

I never believed I would see from under the frown, through the tears or over the enormous challenge of chemotherapy, but I emerged yesterday a very different woman.

Saturday 12 May

We celebrated my birthday – again – tonight with a dinner at our local pub. It was a wonderful evening surrounded by close friends.

Loz made a lovely touching speech and we celebrated once more my birthday and my arrival at this point of the cancer nightmare.

Sunday 13 May

It was an unusual day. During an exhausting whirlwind visit to London, undertaken with renewed vigour, to visit friends, David and Linds, neglected in recent months, visits that are long over-due, I was fed an enormous amount of lovely food to mark the end of the weedkiller – but most memorably of all I was given hair tips by David, whose hair is about one inch long and very spiky. His tips were very useful and I shall be off to search the shops for 'Fudge' (apparently!) which, with its wonderful smell, is 'neither sticky nor tacky but does hold the hair back rather than allowing it to stick up!' So that's lovely!

I must admit that I never thought I would have hair shorter than David.

After being asked by my friends how I was feeling, I noticed during my explanations my mind questioning my words. I found myself explaining such ridiculous thoughts – I note that it hurts when I do that ... my nails hurt when I tap my fingers ... I felt sick for two days ... my thumbnail is rigid ...

There are times when you just have to wonder about one's ability to whinge when quite frankly, you have no right. Get a grip, Pontin – if your nails hurt when you tap them then don't tap them!

Life will feel so much better.

Monday 14 May

Apart from feeling particularly dopey this morning I am entering this week with a renewed vigour, a sense of achievement and a fresh outlook.

Last week I ticked off the second of the four stages of beating this thing – with the diagnosis and mastectomy stage together with the chemotherapy stage now completed, I shall have to focus on the radiotherapy.

Good news! I am trucking on through my usual list of symptoms, which is not quite pleasurable but encouraging at least. However, this morning's exciting discovery is fluff! Yep – fluff! – on my head! This morning I ran my hand over my previously bristly head and to my great excitement I discovered fluff. No longer is it stubbly, like a grumpy old man's beard, but soft and downy. No longer am I the ugly duckling. (No comments from the peanut gallery about being the ugly duckling, thank you!) Quite the show pony now!

All I need are the eyelashes now. They may be the last to fall out but the downside is that they are the last to return.

After further examination I discovered hair on my legs and under my arms, and to my alarm I found myself taking hair advice from a rather thinning big brother – not a state many girls should find themselves in! First David and now Rupes – whatever next?

Wednesday 16 May

Whilst I knew today would come I just wasn't ready for it. My periods have stopped. I was warned that the chemotherapy would probably do this and perhaps bring on the menopause. I had hoped that I had got under the wire on that one, but not so – it appears that my body has managed to fight it off for a while but the inevitable has happened. However, I have done well, apparently, which is a good sign for them to return and for it not being the menopause. Fingers crossed that they return, as every month I have a period means I am still able to have children.

Friday 18 May

Today I was out on the water once again – this time on board with my wonderful husband-to-be. It was fabulous to be sailing with him again, until, to my annoyance, I was walloped on the head with a flogging sheet – and in English for those amongst you who do not speak yacht – I was hit on the head by a rope that was flapping around at great speed at head height.

With one pupil pointing in one direction and the second pointing the other way, I was taken off the boat in a support boat and whisked ashore to be met by an ambulance. With a head injury I was taken to hospital, where I was examined and then eventually released once my pupils behaved. I was so annoyed that it had happened that I asked to be retuned to the yachts – I didn't want to miss anything!

There comes a time when you have to take a step back from the shit from time to time and take a long hard look at what is going on around you. I remain in awe at Rich's continuous love for me throughout this nightmare, and at this point in time I am challenging that love more than ever – one boob, no eyelashes, no hair and now, thanks to today's activities, two black eyes. Sexy, hey?

Sunday 20 May

With the end of Stage Two – the Weedkiller Stage – of this cancer nightmare celebrated privately ten days ago with Rich, I decided that it was a bloody good excuse to have a party to mark this monumental event and thank my friends and family for their unwavering support, so I issued an invitation to a small selection of friends. The support, love and encouragement that both Rich and I have received during the last seven months has been phenomenal and relentless, and I am keen to celebrate and raise a glass with them all – personally, I couldn't have done it without them!

Entitled 'Bugger the Blowfish', the party took place this afternoon with only one condition – everyone had to be sporting an unusual headpiece – oh, and a smile. I can't tell you how varied the collection of goodies that were plonked on their heads has been – underpants, large hysterical wigs, mast-climbing helmets, deer-stalkers, an array of scarves and hats and of course my shocking pink bob wig, which I have taken to wearing whenever a *serious* piece of headwear is required – other than my pink bandana.

Tuesday 5 June

I had a long conversation with my big brother today – not unusual, no, but a conversation I will never forget. He relayed a tale of chitchat between father and son:

'What toy do you have inside your Kinder Egg, Jack?'

On opening his Kinder Egg my nephew, aged seven, pipes up, 'Look Daddy, I have an octopus with cancer!'

Stunned by the response from his son he asks, 'Goodness, Jack, how do you know that the octopus has cancer?'

'Because the octopus is wearing a bandana like Auntie Em!'

His father swiftly explained to him that not all bandana-wearing creatures, great or small, had cancer. Some chose to wear them for fun, like pirates.

Jack listened intensely and then responded, 'So we don't actually know whether the octopus has cancer or not then, Daddy, because he might not have been choosing to wear one and does have cancer after all!'

Ah, the logic of a seven-year-old!

Wednesday 6 June

Cancer is a confusing enough challenge on its own, but my expectations are being blown today. I didn't realise that I would feel worse after chemotherapy than during the process itself. I admit that I have been a very lucky girl – my reaction to chemotherapy has been less challenging physically than I, or anyone around me, was expecting, but to feel tired, fluey and more emotional than ever *after* chemotherapy was not part of the plan.

For seven weeks I am being almost completed ignored by the Southampton Oncology Department, which is bliss. I am currently being given a break from the constant medical prodding, poking and poisoning that I have been experiencing this year and it is lovely! I return to their attentions at the end of June, when I begin the burning process.

Monday 11 June

Simulation Day! Lovely!

Today I went to the radiotherapy centre at Southampton General Hospital for the next stage in my treatment. It is not every patient that takes their own personal radiographer with them – but then I am special!

One of my seven future sisters-in-law, Ranna, is visiting from the other side of the world. I would like to say that she flew over specially for me and my radiotherapy, but I would be lying. She is in fact on holiday here with one of my eight future Australian nieces, Michaela – you see, when I accepted Rich's proposal of marriage I accepted the arrival of seven sisters-in-law, six brothers-in-law, three nephews, eight nieces and three stepchildren. Note to self: always ask questions before accepting offers of any kind.

I felt incredibly guilty taking her with me to this appointment – she has been truly magnificent throughout all this to date, always on the end of the phone for me – but a busman's holiday this was not meant to be. We had made plans for the rest of the day beyond the simulator appointment but I still felt guilty. Needless to say she was her strong supportive and calming self.

It was a truly unpleasant experience – not the meeting with my future sister-in-law but the little oncological outing.

Whilst radiotherapy is painless and non-intrusive, like each and every step in this nightmare it is frightening – for the first time. The fear of the unknown is once again all-encompassing, and I have foolishly enjoyed the freedom of a medical-free diary for the past four glorious weeks.

I spent forty minutes lying topless and very still on a hard cold bed with my left arm up, positioned above my head resting on a cradle. Unable to move, I fixed my gaze on the ceiling and the transfers or stickers that had been placed there, presumably to make the whole experience more pleasant, somehow. Behind my head was the rotating section of the radiation machine or linear accelerator. This section was moved around my body, controlled from a separate chamber, using a series of numbers or coordinates designed to position the rotating drum precisely so that when the beam is released across the surface of my chest, radiating the top layer of skin to eradicate any remaining cancerous cells, it will not penetrate my skin too deeply and therefore will not damage any underlying healthy cells or organs – such as my lungs!

The purpose of today was to establish those coordinates and then to tattoo my chest with two tiny marks – one in the centre of my chest where the first beam would be directed and the second one under my left arm in place for the second beam that would be released from beneath me.

I returned today with shiny new tattoos!

Saturday 16 June

Today my best friend did her Moonwalk for me – or rather she is doing it now. Tonight! As we speak she is pounding the streets of Edinburgh in a fast walk to raise funds for Breast Cancer Care. She and a team of girlfriends have decided to undertake the Moonwalk, which is a twenty-six-mile epic walk – a marathon that will take some eight hours. I am glad I am tucked up in bed.

Monday 2 July

A glorious day indeed! Today, with great excitement, I shaved my legs.

However, I did feel a twinge of betrayal, a little guilty as the little hairs I was so callously shaving off represented life to me. Their re-growth showed that I was alive, fighting back after the termination of the weedkiller treatment – and with all their efforts to show their little faces I smiled delightedly, admired them, and then promptly chopped them off! Charming!

III

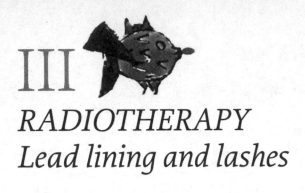

RADIOTHERAPY
Lead lining and lashes

Thursday 5 July 2007

Gone sweeping! When discussing the next stage of treatment in this charming challenge of mine my completely nutty but truly adorable brother suggested that I take a broom with me to my first appointment.

'Why?' I asked, bemused at such an unusual suggestion.

'Because you said that the radiographer's role in this drama is to sweep up any spines that might be left over at the end, and for that you will need a broom!'

Let me explain.

Within the breast and chest wall area tiny microscopic cells may still exist. Cells that have scooted by unnoticed, buried in the skin, so small that the chemotherapy drugs could not find them to cling to. These unseen cells reside in and around the scar area across the chest wall, and the only way to clean up that area is to irradiate it – or 'sweep it' if you are Rupert. For this purpose, this sweeping-up if you will, the consultant will require a broom. Obviously. Bless him!

Anyway, explaining the presence of a broom to my radiographer would be a challenge I could worry about later, I decided as we left home, the little red dustpan brush tucked safely in my bag.

A familiar waiting room met us, clinical and quiet. We

approached the reception, booked in and were directed down some stairs and through a set of doors separating the linear radiation machines from the rest of the world. I noted the doors being heavy, very heavy, serving as a reminder of the intensity of this next round of treatment.

As I looked around the waiting area I recognised many of the faces. They were the familiar faces of the ladies I had come to know during chemotherapy – the Class of 2007. These ladies served as a reminder to me, for I remember when I was sitting and waiting for my first chemotherapy dose all those months ago feeling unusual – like I was the odd one out because I wore nothing on my head (there was no need because my hair was still in abundance as I had yet to receive my first dose of weedkiller) – I remember feeling lucky, relieved almost, as I still resembled a woman, at least when clothed. I also enjoyed the tinge of individuality in a room full of bandanas and hats. From memory there were various garments that adorned the heads of the ladies I was sharing this experience with, their faces sporting a certain gaze and exhibiting a certain comfort that they gained from their headwear. I was aware that I was the new girl on the block and had all of that to come. I had yet to be given my uniform, yet to earn my stripes.

As I moved along the conveyor belt of cancer treatments designed as a belt and braces process to prevent further recurrence of my blowfish I was now sitting in a new building with a new smell but with old faces. The ladies, like me, had moved along that conveyor belt too, ahead of me – and now, in this brightly lit radiography department, the same faces smiled back at me. I was once again the odd one out, but this time in the reverse, this time because I *had* something on my head and they did not – they were sporting very short stylish hair styles – no bandanas, no wigs. How was I ever going to be that brave and shed my bandana, my security blanket, and risk the stares once more? Not me, I could never do that.

I came back to earth with a bump. My name was called, and we moved along the corridor. After a brief, frank and rather rude discussion with a woman in a clinical jacket regarding my treatment and the number of doses we got under way. A rather aggressive and disappointing start to this phase of the treatment which served no purpose other than to make me feel uncomfortable and nervous about what was happening.

I was shown into a large almost empty cold room containing a couple of computer screens, a small changing area and the enormous radiotherapy machine. Looking a little like a bed used for capital punishment, it was familiar to me, as it looked exactly like the simulator I used last month. I hopped on, and after much lifting and moving around of the bed I was left alone. Through a speaker I was asked if I was comfortable. Cold, alone, frightened – but yes, I guess I was comfortable.

I came home today and was forced to face the inevitable. I was told the radiotherapy doses would be daily, and so reluctantly I have had to agree to give up the water for July. I guess it is an excuse for a well-earned rest and finally the ability to admit that I am tired – exhausted actually. I am also now prepared to accept the fact that if I stop working it doesn't mean that the cancer has beaten me – I no longer feel I have to keep moving to keep alive.

Sunday 8 July

With the house empty for a few hours today I sat quietly. I dwelled on my thoughts of last week, my arrival at the radiotherapy clinic, and wondered about my own confidence.

I once swore that I would never learn to feel comfortable in my headwear – the feelings of claustrophobia and frustration. The item only serves as a constant visible reminder that something is wrong. However, over the months it has become a comfort, a security blanket of sorts, for me – and today, when I am so close to shedding the bandana look, admittedly in exchange for a rather unusual, if a little pixie-like, lesbian look that I have taken on, I battle with my confidence. How am I ever going to leave the house 'naked' from the neck up?

Whilst I truly believe I have reached my limit of constantly wearing something on my head I am clearly not as comfortable as I thought I was. My darling long-suffering husband-to-be has shown a different way of dealing with this particular stage of the challenge – instead of encouraging me to shed my 'blanket' he just says 'that's great, you are nearly there' – which initially was not helping because I need to be pushed at times, but the more I thought about this response the more I felt the pressure I had placed on me to go 'naked' was not there at all. 'You have to walk before you can run, Em,' he said. 'Get comfortable at home before you face the world – there's no hurry!'

So that is what I decided to. And after first checking the garden and the front path for errant bodies that might surprise me I became bold and took it off! It felt wonderful and odd at the same time. I spent some time staring into the mirror at myself and then suddenly – there was knock at the door. Oh my God, who could that be? Had someone seen me through the window? I flapped around looking for my bandana, running up and down the stairs like a crazy woman, but I couldn't find it – where on earth had I put it? Again the knock at the door. Unable to find my 'blanket' I grabbed the nearest thing and opened the door. The postman – poor chap – tried not to look amused at this apparition that stood before him. He must have seen some things in his time, but this? He was faced with a woman sporting a pair of red shorts, a T-shirt with the logo 'unforgettable bird' blazed across a very odd-shaped chest, a pair of flip-flops with white daisies on them, all topped off with a beautiful pink woolly hat. And before you ask, it was the first thing I could grab from the hat stand next to the front door. This was, after all, not a glamorous time in my life.

With the postman safely on his way I removed the woollen number and shot out into the garden for a quick run around – because I could. When I stood still, I could feel the wind blowing my hair, just gently, sending a tingle down my neck – it was bloody brilliant.

Monday 9 July

The fiasco that is my fight against this cancer continued today. Mind you, after the missed diagnosis at the outset some nine months ago and the unfortunate experience of witnessing a cardiac arrest during my first dose of chemotherapy, why I am surprised that radiotherapy has not gone off without a hitch, I do not know!

With Rich unable to work from home today I was alone for a treatment appointment for the first time since all this began. I wandered into the radiotherapy clinic – a fresh week and a fresh attitude, I thought to myself. I can do this! Clutching my little piece of paper displaying my barcode – a series of numbers that is unique to me and my cancer – I strolled into the reception and ambled down the steps to the left, through the huge heavy doors, and proceeded to the registration machine. After 'clocking in' I grabbed the nearest magazine to act as a form of escapism and sank myself into the chair, burying my head in the world of Victoria Beckham and her latest escapades. I sat for many minutes, pretending I was anywhere but here. Time passed and I became uncomfortable and began to fidget. The arrival, and subsequent disappearance, of many of my counterparts helped to exaggerate the delay. Something was wrong. Oh God something was wrong!

Like a child playing hide and seek, tucked down behind the sofa yet desperate to see if anyone was looking for her, I gingerly raised my head at an acute angle, peered under my heavy eye-lids and saw a white coat walking towards me with a determined gait. The delay was wrong – something was wrong!

Sadly, I was right.

The White Coat was the dreadful creature who met us on Day One. My mind was spinning, negative thoughts filled my head. What had they discovered when they took that picture of my lung on Friday? The cancer had spread, I was sure. Heaving a great sigh I raised my head, and my game, and looked her in the eye.

She approached me, sat down and delivered a statement in what I can only describe as the most inappropriate fashion, the likes of which I had yet to receive in this debacle. She then got up to leave, denying me the opportunity to respond or to question what she had said.

Stunned, I stood straight and steady and put my hand on her arm to stop her leaving. I asked her to repeat the comment, to which she responded, 'Oh, you are clearly not going to let go of this, are you?' and suggested I follow her into a private room, muttering from four steps ahead of me that she was not supposed to tell me the full details of what had happened.

I followed Little Miss White Coat down the corridor, into a room, and sat quietly whilst she explained, in as little detail as she could get away with, that they had given me the wrong dose and I would have to start my radiotherapy again. 'We are not supposed to tell you,' she said – that was the part that stunned me most. Why? I thought. Why not tell me? Such a serious treatment for such a serious disease, and a patient is not supposed to be told of any discrepancies or errors? Surely that could not be right.

The delay was because they were trying to locate my consultant radiologist, to advise him of the error and confirm the new programme with the new timings and dosages before beginning the treatment again. As if satisfied that she had done her job appropriately, and once again giving me no chance to absorb and respond to her comments, she got up to leave.

I concluded that the white coat and I were not going to get on well. Two meetings and two arguments did not bode well for the next fortnight!

As you can imagine I found this wholly unsatisfactory and I gave her both barrels, starting with the appalling manner in which she had first spoken to me and moving on to the disgraceful way in which she was handling the situation today. I tried to explain to her that it was frightening to be told that there is a problem with the treatment. Were the levels of radiation already given to me going to harm me? I tried to explain that I had questions that I wanted to ask.

After further discussion I discovered that, whilst the consultant radiologist had signed and approved my dose, it was in fact *she* who was responsible for this latest error. That it was in fact our Miss White Coat who was responsible for the programming of the dose into the machine which delivered the radiation. Not a simple task, as the figures and corrections involved rival that of celestial navigation. Nonetheless, as with celestial navigation, errors in the calculations can produce results that can be just as disastrous. Her aggression began to make sense to me. It was her error and she was embarrassed.

We spoke – no, I spoke – for a few minutes, and I believe that she was left knowing in no uncertain terms how I was feeling. I challenged her to imagine herself in my shoes, to imagine being told that there was a problem with the treatment she was undergoing, a problem that appeared to me to derive from the photograph of the lung that was taken the previous Friday as I left as no-one had taken the time to tell me otherwise. I challenged her to imagine what it was like to be chastised for having the nerve to believe that I had a right to ask a question, any question, in relation to what was going on with *my* body! The fear, the panic and the anxiety that race through one's body when someone wearing a white coat tells you that there is a problem is all-encompassing. I suggested that she would feel just the same as I did that day and yet she would be streets ahead of patients like myself as she was trained and understood what the machines and treatments are all doing.

She apologised! I stared. She left.

———

I mused that with every dream team there must be an anti. My wonderful oncologist Dr Symonds came as a welcome relief after the gruff character that was my consultant breast surgeon. My dream ward sister who took so much care and time with me that night immediately after my mastectomy came on the back of my run-in with the registrar and his black pen. My angels in the chemotherapy clinic, Jenny and Elaine, were a blessing after the horrifically impatient nurse whom I had the misfortune to experience one day and who frankly should learn to understand the fear of just what it means to a person to have poison pumped directly into her veins, cold and thick.

My wonderful breast care nurse, big and bubbly, with warmth in her huge smile, was very supportive and a welcome sight after the pinched expressions showing lack of patience and under-standing of some of her colleagues. And finally my radiogra-phers, who settle me into my machine and deliver the dose, who explain each and every move they make, the moves the machine makes and my expected feelings and symptoms, they come as a welcome antidote to the White Coat!

I conclude today with the thought that bedside manner is not a dedicated topic of discussion in the medical degrees of today. Patience, tolerance and understanding clearly cannot be taught. They are traits that some medical professionals are unfortunate-ly not blessed with – still, you cannot have it all.

Tuesday 10 July

I listened patiently to my consultant radiologist as he spoke at length, explaining the error of dose and reasons behind it. He then tried desperately to justify the White Coat's attitude and rudeness of yesterday. He failed.

To me it was not justifiable.

I proceeded to correct him on the events that took place, and from the resultant expressions on his face I would suggest that he was unaware of the level of rudeness that had been afforded to me. Whilst I accept that we are all human and errors happen, her attitude was no error but plain thoughtlessness, a complete failure to understand a cancer patient's position.

However, he calmed my nerves and reassured me that no

damage had been done due to the incorrect dosage, and we moved forward with a plan for the rest of my treatment.

It is true to say that I do not get this radiotherapy business, though. You see it neither touches nor shows any form of intrusion on your body.

Lying motionless on a table in a cool, dark room, naked from the waist up with your arm raised and secured above your head, with the mutterings of the radiographers and the buzzing of the machine as it is moved electronically around your body the only sounds to break the deathly silence. Despite the presence of the radiographers whose company I shared, the feelings of loneliness and vulnerability consume – a very odd experience.

It is true that when someone says 'don't move' the first thing you want to do is move. 'Breathe normally, Miss Pontin' results in the instant desire to sigh, heaving the chest and upsetting the green laser lines lying across my body that measure the angles that are vital to this treatment, the angles that measure the area to be irradiated and that reduce the damage to the lung.

I have spent the first three doses lying motionless, barely daring to breathe so as to reduce the movement of my chest, listening to the machine – counting the seconds that the radiation is penetrating my chest and willing the time to pass so that I could leave that room. Today, however, clearly ready for answers, I plucked up the courage to ask what was happening. What the noises meant, why the need for so much movement of a machine that requires such immobility from the patient and the reasons why they no longer visited me in my room between the two doses and simply controlled the exercise from their antechamber, which represented a position of safety. To me their visit between the two doses signalled that I was not alone, that they had not forgotten me and that all was well.

Each of the two doses administered, one either side of my body, is designed to accommodate the shape of my chest wall, skimming the surface of my skin to reduce unnecessary damage to my lung with the gel blanket absorbing the depth the beam is trying to travel.

'Buzzing', 'wedges' and 'cooking' were words that explain my experience, the visits of which are reducing in number. Eleven to go!

Oh – today's top tip. Do not take an electronically marked car-park ticket into a radiation room – it will not work afterwards.

Wednesday 11 July

Another day, another dose, another learning curve.

I wandered confidently into the radiography clinic today – early. I had plans to sit and write my thoughts and feelings before my appointment. I find my words flow more easily when surrounded by the circumstances. I clocked in and made a cup of tea and began to write.

Needless to say, things change. I was called – early! – God forbid! Such a shock was it that I mentioned it to my radiographer. She too was a little unnerved.

There was an air of confidence about me today and a certain familiarity that breeds a level of comfort in these unusual surroundings. We got under way and I lay, deep in thought, whilst the girls relayed the figures to one another, the figures that correlated to my dose, and moved my bed around accordingly. Within seconds they had left the room for the safety of their control room and I was left, alone with my thoughts once again.

Left side – first buzz – the subsequent retraction of the wedge – second buzz. No sign of my radiographers, who had clearly decided to stay in their antechamber, and so we continued. On to the right side – first buzz – and just waiting for the usual retraction of the wedge when the lights came on. Why?

That was wrong, the lights were wrong. They were not meant to come on. My comfort zone was feeling shaken. I reasoned with myself that a wrong button had been pressed in the control room but the panic had begun – if they could press a light-switch button by mistake then they could press any button by mistake.

I wanted to move but I dared not – I waited until the sound of the retraction of the wedge rang out and I began to breathe heavily, moving my chest up and down, knowing I only had a few seconds to do this before I had to find calm again otherwise the radiation beam would penetrate my skin too deeply and deliver a dangerous dose to my lung. I had to find calm.

Never did find the answer to the light issue.

Thursday 12 July

I was angry when I woke up this morning. Angry with this whole episode. Clearly today was going to be frustrating – a day when I try and understand and fail. I can have a fiery temper, and in an effort to elevate my mood I went for a wander down on 'my' beach – my escape from reality and a place where I can let off steam.

I spent some time just watching the water, lapping up and down on the shore. Trying to find calm. I had to go to the clinic again today and I didn't want to be angry all day.

Sunday 15 July

I took part in the Race for Life today flanked by two future brides-maids, Jen and Rach, on either side of me. And with front-row spots alongside a dear friend, yachtswoman Dee Caffari, who is patron of the charity Sail 4 Cancer, we counted down with 10,000 other women to the start. The nervous tension that builds on a start line grew, the tension that I remember and love from my running days – 10, 9, 8 – nearly there – 3, 2, 1 and we were off – a 5 km run through the streets of Southampton on a beautiful Sunday morning in July – how wonderful.

I had a ball – I love running and it was such a beautiful day. However, after 3 km I needed to walk a while – I counted one thousand paces and then started to run again. I crossed the line in just under 30 minutes and should have been delighted but personally I considered that I had failed as I was unable to run the whole distance, and for someone like me who is a runner I found this frustrating. But some things are better in perspective, aren't they – my friends were impressed that I entered at all and ran as much as I did. I ought to have been grateful really. Clearly I was a lucky girl to be able to undertake such a physical challenge at all during this cancer nightmare with chemicals, poisons and radiotherapy – I wound my neck in almost immediately.

Monday 16 July

I paid the price for my run yesterday. I was lucky enough to be on the start line for this event alongside the record-breaking yachts-woman Dee and sporting my familiar and very recognisable pink bandana (which had still not been off my head for longer than it takes to wash the thing) with the television cameras broadcasting the faces of our little group around the television area of the south coast.

On my arrival at the hospital for the first of my five daily doses this week I was met by stern glances from the radiographers, who were unimpressed, if a little amazed, that I had undertaken such a strenuous activity whilst undergoing radiation to the chest. It is without doubt the most trouble I have felt in since I started this cancer rollercoaster!

Friday 20 July

We headed north this afternoon – destination north-west and the borders of the Lake District to visit my dearest Gilly and her family. The road trip started well until we hit Oxford and then all hell broke loose. Parts of England had been engulfed in torrential rain, the likes of which I have never seen before, in a beautiful band from east to west across the country separating those in the south from their friends north of Oxford. Roads were closed and motorways backed up in the most horrendous traffic jams.

After two hours of battling to get past the backlog of traffic Rich and I returned to Hamble and reported in to Destination Briggs. Reluctantly we called off the road trip and promised to be there by coffee-time tomorrow.

Saturday 21 July

Dawn broke and we set off – ridiculously early frankly but nevertheless no traffic – bound for the Lakes. There was a party arranged for all those who took part in the Moonwalk in June.

As promised, we arrived in time for coffee. I shot upstairs, showered, dressed and with my pink bandana in place I started downstairs to join the party. However, the bandana was irritating me, slipping and itching. My hair was doing its best to grow back, and making a very good job of it, but I still looked decidedly dodgy and I still preferred to hide behind the familiar cover of my pink 'hat'.

I returned to the bedroom and frustratingly retied the thing at least twice before Gilly appeared. She could see I was frustrated and annoyed, and with the encouragement and strength of this wonderful friend I took the thing off and stared in the mirror. So far I think I had managed to get away with looking like a slightly trendy sailor, but now I looked like a cancer patient. Together we made the decision to go downstairs and face the music, brave the stares. The room was filled with people who had never met me before and who therefore did not know what I looked like with hair, and this proved to be easier than I thought – they had nothing to judge me against and so just smiled at me and continued to drink and chat – perfect!

Rich hugged me and Gilly cried – but overall a good decision.

Thursday 26 July

Feeling a little less anxious about the prospect of being set free from my oncological strings. The butterflies still fluttered today, though, in anticipation of tomorrow I guess.

Friday 27 July

Pink, brown, flaky – done! That's what I have to look forward to over the next month. Apparently I'm cooked. No more random burning sessions of my chest. It's all over.

I've been set free and was told that my skin, which was rapidly turning pink, would turn brown – just like sunburn – then flaky – lovely!

Today we put a tick in box number three – the radiotherapy treatment. I must admit that it was okay really. I had heard all sorts of horror stories that, by the end of the radiotherapy, I would be sleeping twenty out of twenty-four hours a day.

It was unintrusive and painless. Just a little worrying, as they are aiming a radioactive beam directly at your carefully protected vital breathing apparatus – the heart and lungs. However, with the help of a whole host of numbers and just a little bit of science they appear to have missed all the relevant parts. My chest is marked by a beautiful red square showing where I have slowly been cooked over the past three weeks, which will reduce in shine and colour, but otherwise all seems to be well.

Saturday 28 July

Today was wedding day! Not mine but that of my friends Giles and Verity. I was required to look smart. One thing I have been able to do over the past six months is to hide behind being scruffy. As a sailor who spends most of her time in jeans, sailing kits or sportswear I have been able to shy away from looking smart. Not today.

No, my sailing foulies would not be acceptable. I rummaged through my wardrobe and settled on a white trouser suit with a halter-neck top that provided room for my prosthesis. For my head I selected a black woollen pashmina which looked great but was very, very hot indeed. It had decided to be warm and sunny today and we were about to spend the afternoon sitting in a large marquee. However, I was able to take the jacket off and let off some steam.

I counted my eyelashes this morning too and decided that it was mascara day. Looking like a girl again, and with just a touch of elegant sophistication about me, I hoped, I headed off to the church with Rich and my parents.

Monday 13 August

After a very hectic Cowes Week regatta, we set sail today on the infamous Fastnet Race. The 650-mile course starts from Cowes on the Isle of Wight and takes the fleet along the beautiful Dorset and Devon coast and around the tip of Cornwall before racing up to the Fastnet Rock sitting just off the southern tip of Ireland and back again, rounding Land's End to finish just off Plymouth.

This race became infamous in 1979 when a huge low-pressure system charged through the fleet with disastrous consequences, with many yachts abandoned and many lives lost. Let us hope this year is slightly less challenging – although with the race start delayed for the first time in its history due to gale-force wind warnings I am not hopeful.

I have competed in this biennial race twice previously and on both occasions the weather has been very light and incredibly frustrating, resulting in anchors being deployed to prevent many yachts in the fleet from being carried backwards by the current, unsupported by the lack of wind.

We finally got under way twenty-four hours late, and with the fleet beating into the strong head winds blowing from the south-west we anticipated a hairy first leg to Land's End. We were not disappointed! This was my first race since the diagnosis and the completion of the treatment and I felt like a new woman today. Not chained to the medics and finally being allowed to travel offshore for the first time in months – I felt elated despite the battering we were getting. The bow was a very wet place to be but I didn't care!

Friday 17 August

Well, we are home again after a very disappointing race from which we had to retire. The heavy winds took their toll on much of the fleet, with only some forty entrants completing the course. A nasty year out there on the water – but that is yacht racing for you. There is always 2009.

I just hope I fare better in the two remaining races of the year that I am competing in – a transatlantic to the Caribbean and the Sydney to Hobart yacht race – another feisty race with a heavy history!

Monday 20 August

Rich and I flew off to the USA today to see his children. I have not seen them since Christmas and I am very aware that I will look different to them – I barely have any hair and look decidedly like a boy.

We have shared my cancer with them – Rich went out to visit them in the spring – both face to face and on the phone and they have been fantastic. They have a cousin in Australia who has battled leukaemia, and so baldness, chemotherapy and hospitals are all familiar territory for these small children.

Sunday 26 August

I have the energy of a crazy woman these days! Not sure why but possibly because I have been handed my life back and am not sure how long I have got with it. So I am doing everything at a hundred miles an hour. This is not unusual for me but is probably exhausting for Rich. I am conscious that I cannot sit still, and I assume that as time passes I will relax a little – but not yet. Hell no! I have things I need to do and I need to do them all now! You never know what is round the corner, and if this thing comes back I want to be ready.

Wednesday 29 August

We had a wonderful time in the United States with the children. We spoke of life together and our future as a family. It was a carefree break after the tension of the past nine months. We spent time on the river kayaking, on the trampoline and playing games – it was a wonderful time and the relief clearly showed in Rich and me.

For the first time I was looking at these children who were now about to become my stepchildren and play an enormous part in my life, a life I was still not sure I was going to have. However, it was wonderful to get to know them and spend some time with them.

Wednesday 19 September

We received some devastating news this morning. A woman who is very close to our hearts and who played a vital role in our lives at the beginning of this nightmare has herself just been diagnosed with breast cancer.

It was thanks in no small part to this woman and her support for two people she did not know at all some ten and a half months ago when I received 'that call' that we have been able to believe that there could be a silver lining to what then loomed as a very dark cloud. As she and her husband quite rightly pointed out to us, the situation was not as bleak as human nature would have us believe. We are delighted to learn, though, that she will not have to undergo chemotherapy.

Sunday 23 September

We travelled to France this weekend to spend some time with two of Rich's Australian friends, Bob and Jos, who have a beautiful old stone house on the river in a stunning French village. For a Francophile like me it was heaven.

The Rugby World Cup is being hosted by France this year and we have been lucky enough to be able to get tickets for one of the matches – and so today I was forced to sit in the Australia camp in the Stade de la Mosson in Montpellier at the 2007 Rugby World Cup pool match of Australia vs Fiji. If I had had my way I would have been supporting Fiji, but as my hosts were Australian, my husband-to-be is Australian, and the other friends with us were Australian, I was forced to play the role of Australian Sheila for the day and sported a green and gold jersey and was seen at some point with the Australian flag draped around my shoulders. Clearly I was not myself!

Tuesday 2 October

Today is Rich's fortieth birthday. Dates and events are fast approaching as life moves on and I am aware that I am actually at those events. It is wonderful to be celebrating his birthday.

I organised the best present ever – today England played Australia in the 2007 Rugby World Cup! Now that took some organising, I can tell you.

After a gift-laden breakfast in bed a very proud Australian wandered downstairs in his fancy green and gold rugby jersey content in the knowledge that his home team were going to do him proud on this day of all days.

With the sour taste of the 2003 Rugby World Cup final still in his mouth (on home turf too) I think Rich was expecting to spend much of today gloating. Stupid boy!

To celebrate his birthday I organised a party which was to continue long into the night after the match – regardless of who won! A sea of white rugby jerseys started to arrive just after lunch and in time to grab a beer before the start. A noisy start was punctuated with the call for more beer, and as the match progressed the once deafening vocals with the Australian twang began to weaken as our English lads did us proud on the pitch. Conspicuous by his absence as the final whistle blew, I knew he was in for a long night.

This is revenge for the episode in France. Oh how the mighty have fallen!!

Wednesday 10 October

Today was my first three-monthly checkup.

After being fed weedkiller religiously for four months, radiated until I was sure I would glow in the dark (never mind showing up on radar), stripped of one particularly vital asset – oh and my hair and dignity too – today I shouted from the superhighway rooftop the news that I have blown my blowfish to kingdom come!

I asked what the process was from here onwards. It was explained that I have to monitor myself over the next three months and report any consistent pain or ache – but the key word was consistent. As I have been told before, cancer patients will continue to suffer the same aches and pains non-cancer patients get – colds, muscle twinges etc – and it is important that I monitor them and report in with any concerns. The truth is they are always at the end of the phone but I must admit to feeling very anxious when I discovered that the checkups contained nothing other than a poke around the chest and underarm area together with questions about my health over the past few months.

I must admit I could not have seen this day that dismal moment last year when the doctors dropped the bomb – but somehow we have managed to get here, and I would love to thank Team Blowfish, without whom I could not have survived, and I will. Their love and words of support and encouragement have been invaluable.

It seems only fitting that I should be given the all clear during October – Breast Cancer Awareness Month and almost a year to the day since my diagnosis.

I was described today by a dear friend of mine as 'one tough old bird' – a compliment, I believe?

I was told that if I could beat this on determination alone then I would have won months ago. If enthusiasm and grim determination were a winning combination then many people would win, but I feel I have – today at least.

Thursday 11 October

After the dust settles, the chaos calms and the panic and fear subside, when the heart stops racing and reduces to a gentle gallop – it is then that you realise that you are still standing.

I no longer consider myself unlucky – rather, I am lucky. I had passed people whose treatment had not been successful and whom I had come to rely upon. Their faces had become safe and familiar. However, familiarity breeds contempt, and there is a danger in assuming that all will be well. For me it is, to date at least, but for many their challenges continue.

Conscious of the 'easy ride' I have had throughout my treatment, I remain painfully aware that the less debilitating physical reaction I had to the chemotherapy poisons is unusual, and a blessing, and has made my battle that much more manageable. True, I was convinced at stages that they were giving me the wrong drugs and so questioned my body's response – but, reassured, I have learnt that my body is just more robust than I thought.

They caught my cancer in time and were able to remove or chase down all the cells. I did not develop lymphoedema, a condition connected with the removal of the lymph glands resulting in the permanent swelling of the arm where the glands were removed from. This is a horrible and constant reminder to those that do suffer from lymphoedema of the nightmare that is their breast cancer. I showed no debilitating reactions to my chemotherapy, no sickness or weakness, and was therefore able to continue my life, to continue to do my very physical and challenging job as a skipper, for which I shall be eternally grateful.

I read an interview recently with the Australian pop sensation Kylie Minogue, a fellow breast cancer survivor, who said (*Glamour*, October 07) 'You don't forget – you move forward ... Your body and muscles have a memory of the way it was when you were sick and there are definitely times when I float back to that place. Times when I experience a pain in the arm or chest and think – Oh God, No please!'

———

It is easy to refer to myself as a cancer survivor, which I am – to date, anyway. But it is not the sum of who I am, it is a part of me.

After my earlier reflections I tried to focus on today's events. Today was very important to me, as today Rich and I went for our first appointment with the surgeon who will be performing my right prophylactic mastectomy followed by the bilateral reconstruction.

I am now entering the exciting stage, the process of being 'rebuilt'. After being categorically destroyed – and being left to slowly watch my body fall apart around my ears – the hair loss, the eyelashes and the boob – I now feel like I have turned a corner.

He explained the various options available to me, and after a cursory glance at my naked upper body he began to explain the future with two boobs once again.

Reconstructive surgery is available in several forms, but as a slim, small-breasted female there appeared to be just one suitable option to me – the latissimus dorsi flap reconstruction. With little fat on my back and only a small breast to replace, it was the perfect option.

There are many considerations for potential latissimus dorsi flap patients. My breast reconstruction is very important to me. The loss of my breast translated into a diminished sense of femininity and a loss of confidence and the feeling of normality, and I was keen to learn all about this procedure that would return all those feelings to me, completing the circle and providing closure for this little adventure of mine.

The reconstructive surgeon advised me that should I consider a latissimus dorsi flap reconstruction I would be left with scarring at the donor site on the back as well as on my chest. He also confirmed that it is major surgery and therefore the recovery period would be significant.

He explained that the latissimus dorsi is the long muscle that runs beneath the armpit and diagonally across the back – when you raise your arm, the muscle can be felt along the side of the rib cage. Because of this muscle's proximity to the chest area, utilising tissue from this region for breast reconstruction after a mastectomy is a popular technique among cosmetic surgeons. Additionally, the muscle and skin flap can remain attached to its natural blood supply, making the procedure less complex and reducing the risk of rejection or complications.

I was advised that the procedure would take about five to six hours.

He proceeded to explain the pluses and minuses of latissimus dorsi flap reconstruction, to include the potential temporary loss of strength in my back, a difference in colour of the skin on my back to the skin on my chest and the risks of breast asymmetry.

After much discussion it was agreed that my name would be put on the list for surgery as soon as possible. I had always promised myself that I would not go down the aisle with one boob, and with the wedding arranged for July next year and the first available date for an operation showing as February, to be followed by what could be a six-month complete recovery period, we knew we did not have time on our hands.

A truly successful day I think.

Sunday 14 October

I went to church today and during Holy Communion I prayed. I am not particularly religious – though I was christened and confirmed and, as a teenager, taught Sunday school at my village church – but for some reason I decided I wanted to pray today.

Mostly I gave thanks – for sparing me. One year ago it was a common feeling through my family that there was perhaps no God and if there was, he was not very friendly at all after the stunt he had just pulled. However, throughout this whole episode I have wondered regularly if he in fact saved my life, saved me from myself. We go back to the first question of why? Why me?

Well, I have learnt that I will never be able to answer that.

I know, I know – I should have been praying for something a little less selfish but I wasn't asking for anything, taking his time and his efforts away from those who needed him more, I was simply thanking him. True I wanted his time, just for a minute, I wanted him to listen and hear my words – but not to do anything – just to smile.

On the brighter side, it has forced me to have a make-over. A new hairstyle, and for the first time in twenty years I experienced life without mascara, or the blue/black eyelash tint I took to aged seventeen. (Well, as a blonde it was absolutely necessary if I wanted to look a little less like someone who had been throwing up all night!)

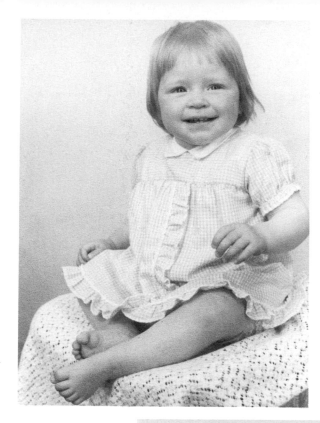

◄ Aged 1 in 1971.

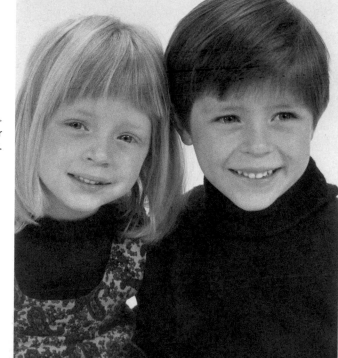

► With my brother Rupert.

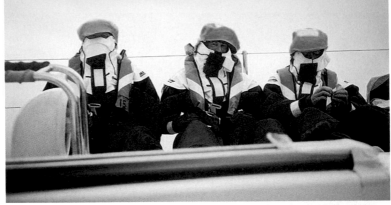

▲ On the rail – my first
transatlantic race, 2002.

►

Mid-watch, exhausted, during the
same race (red glow from condensation
on the lens, not Ready Brek).

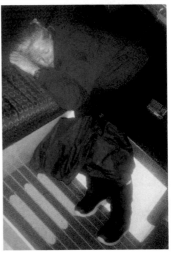

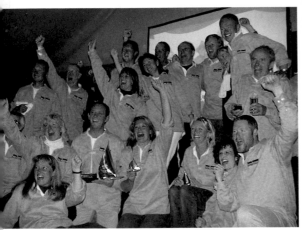

◄ We win first place –
at the prizegiving, 2002.

With Jen, leaving the Kiel
Canal, Germany, 2003.
▼

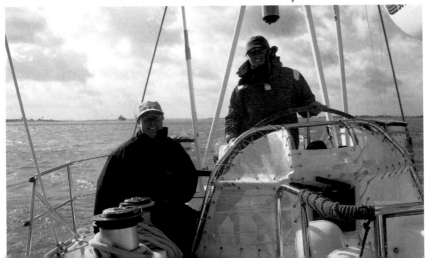

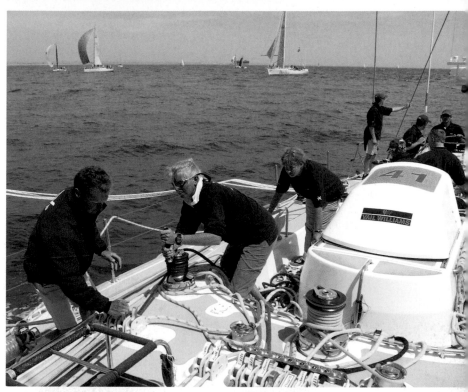

▲ Grinding to first place in the Round-the-Island race, 2003.

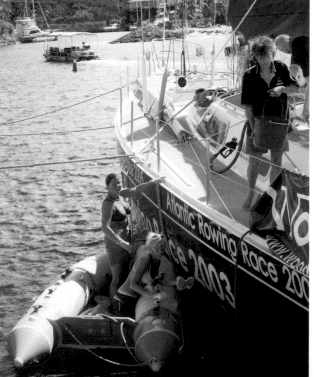

◀ Hard at work, hull-cleaning, Barbados 2003 (we didn't row there).

Sailing *BG Spirit* in the Solent in 2004. This yacht was a competitor in Gobal Challenge 2004, but for the race itself I was on a rival yacht: *Me to You*.

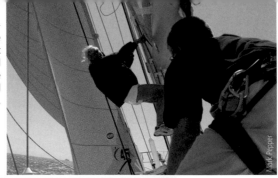

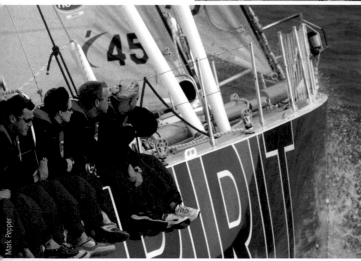

◄ On the rail – *BG Spirit*, 2004.

In the snake pit – *BG Spirit*, 2004.
▼

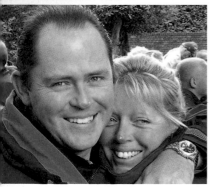

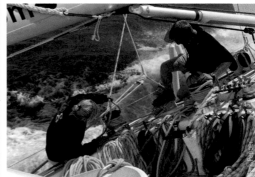

▲
With brother Rupert before the start of the Global Challenge race, October 2004. The blue noses are thanks to my team's sponors, Carte Blanche, designers of Tatty Teddy greetings cards.

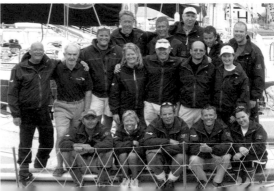

The *Me to You* Global Challenge team at Southampton, August 2004.

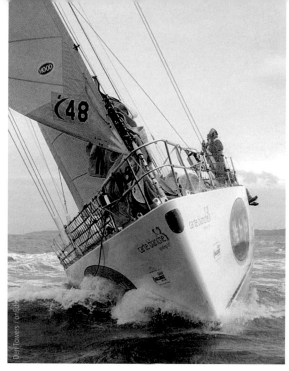

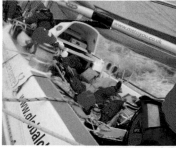

◀ *Me to You* gets going, Global Challenge 2004.

Leg 1 – en route to Buenos Aires. ▼

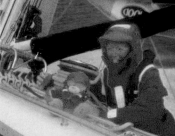

With Tatty Teddy, in work togs – ▶

– and out (it wasn't all hard work). ▼

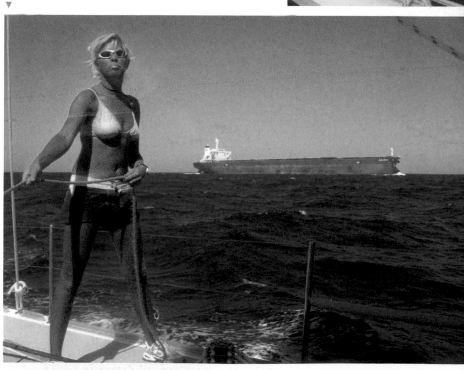

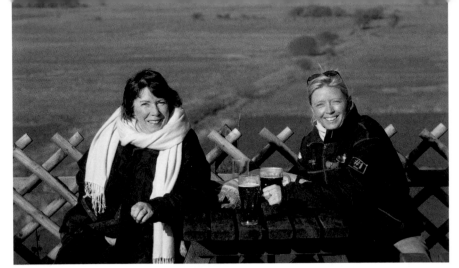

▲ With Mummy at home in Sussex, 2005.

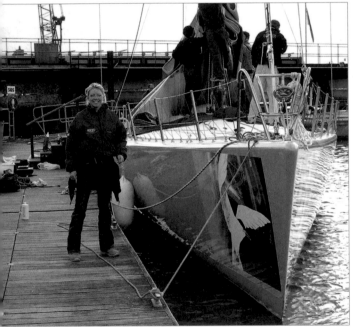

◀ Alongside the Volvo 60 racing yacht *Pindar*, skippered by my friend Loz, en route to the Centenary Newport Bermuda yacht race, April 2006 .

▶ Working as skipper, in October 2006, just before the diagnosis.

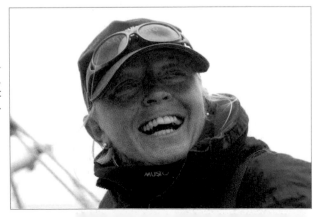

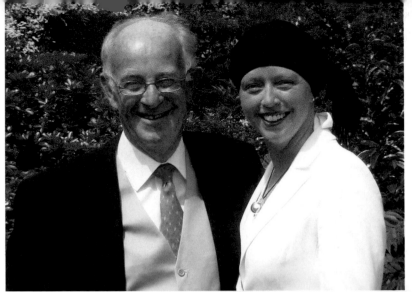

▲
With Daddy in smart headwear for a friend's wedding.

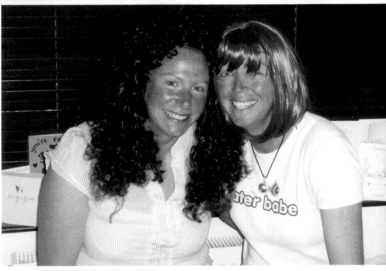

▲ With friend Rach, at my Bugger the Blowfish party in May 2007.

◀ Chemotherapy finished, July 2007.

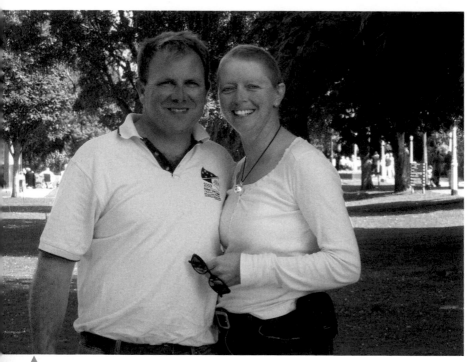

July 2007, with Rich –

– and with Gilly.

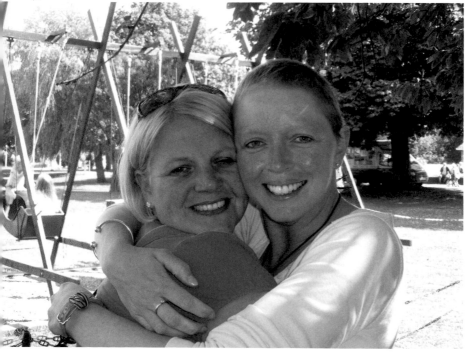

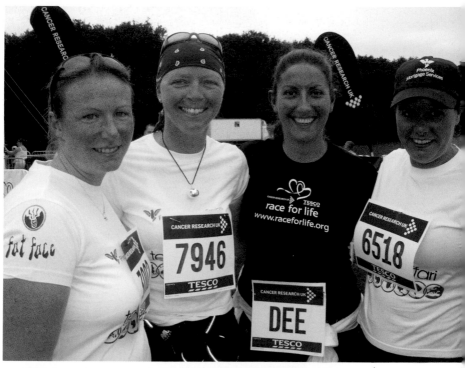

Rach, me, Dee and Jen – Race for Life, July 2007.

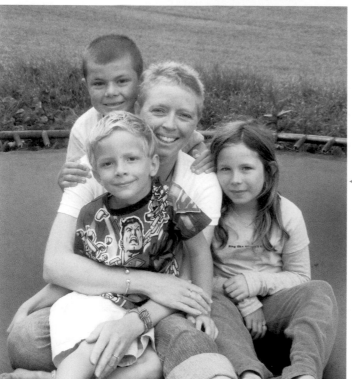

With my soon-to-be stepchildren, Han, Dan and Nick, in the USA, August 2007.

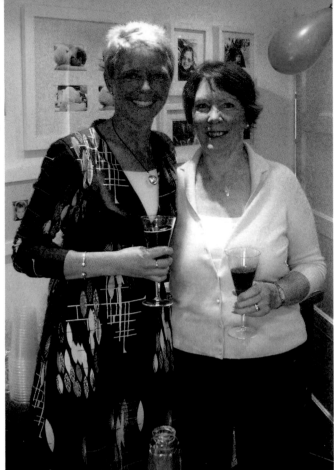

With Mummy ▶
at Rich's 40th,
October 2007.

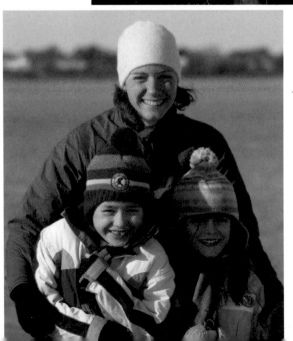

◀ My sister Kate with
the twins, Jack and
Georgia.

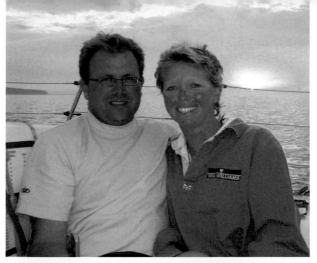

◄ With Rich at the Sydney to Hobart race, 2007.

With the crew of *Kioni*, in Sydney before the Sydney to Hobart race, 2007.
▼

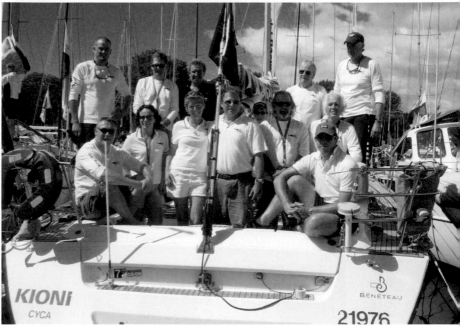

March 2008 - (left) the results of the left mastectomy, and (right) after the prophylactic right mastectomy and reconstructive surgery.
▼

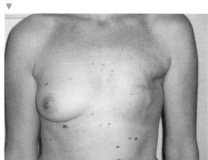
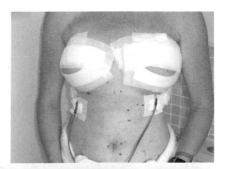

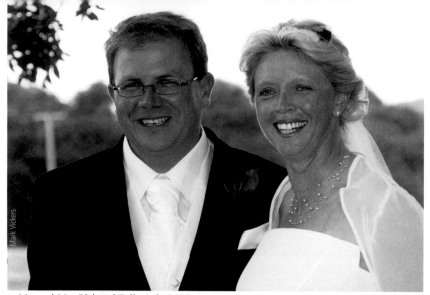

▲ Mr and Mrs Richard Falk, July 2008.

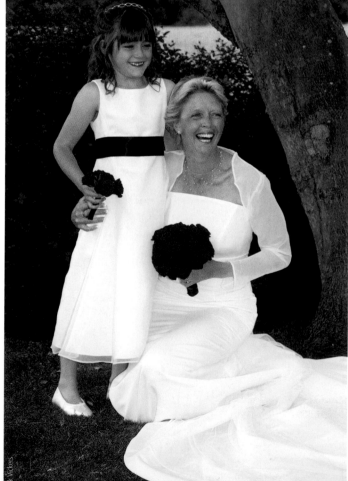

► With my niece Georgia on my wedding day.

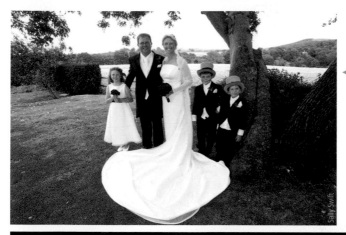

◄ Family Falk: Han, Rich, Em, Dan and Nick.

Flying off on honeymoon by helicopter.
▼

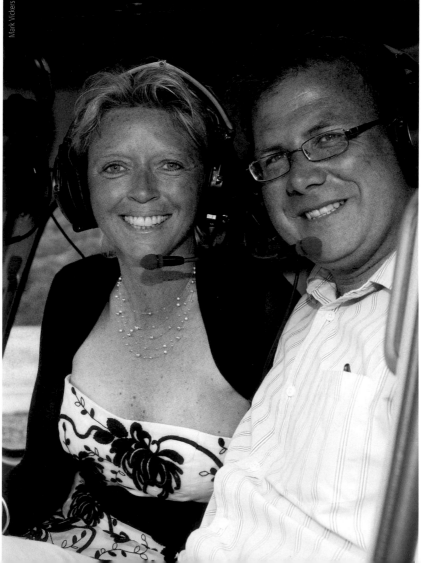

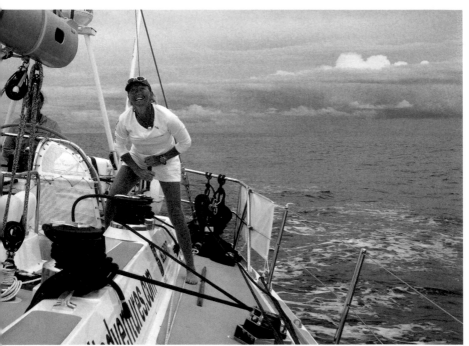

▲ Winching – ARC transatlantic race, 2008.

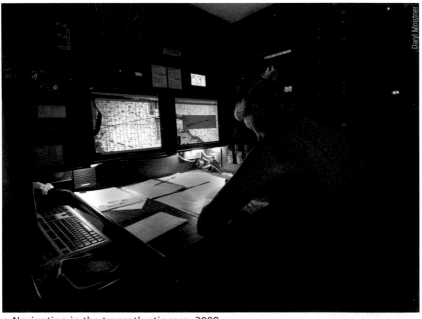

▲ Navigating in the transatlantic race, 2008.

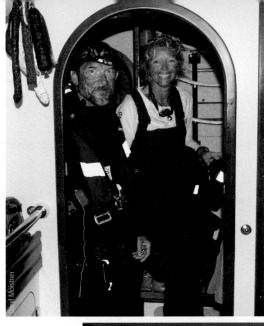

◄ Midnight watch change, transatlantic race, 2008.

Lucky we had GPS; using a sextant with sunglasses can put you out several degrees of latitude, but once a celebrity ...
▼

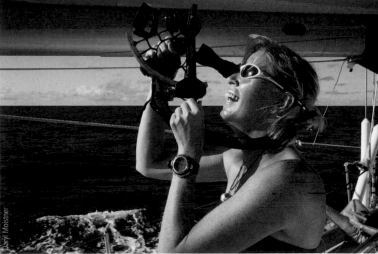

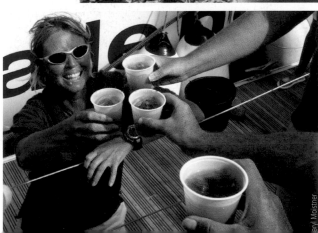

◄ Transatlantic race finish – St Lucia, 2008.

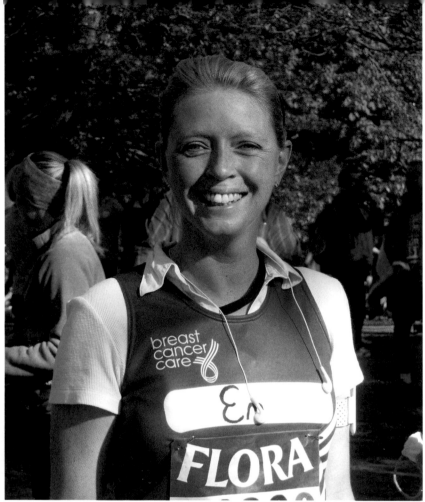

▲ At the start of the London Marathon, April 2009.

▼ Em and Rich, April 2009.

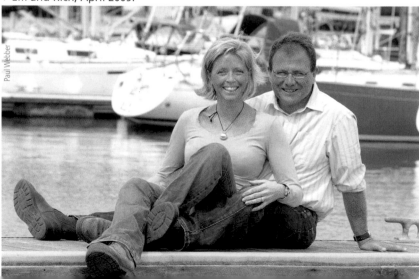

It has forced me to address my fears. A long overdue smear brought good news, my first eye test in eight years and a drop in cholesterol have all been subsidiary outcomes. Perhaps it has forced me to address my body – an awesome machine that I have, to date, been terrified of as I have never really understood it.

In an attempt to keep fighting, and in an effort to hold on to the strength needed, it is vital that I hold a true belief in myself and hold in focus a future for myself. Even though I have been set free from the constant gaze of the medical team I still feel very vulnerable. I still get my wobbles – particularly around the build-up to my periodic checks. They will never go away. They may pale with time, I guess, but I don't expect them to ever really go. I try daily to drive forward to reach each new goal I set myself, and my first is to skipper that transatlantic yacht race that I missed a year ago when I received my diagnosis. I will complete that in November. My second goal is my wedding day – our wedding day – set for 12 July 2008.

Tuesday 23 October

We went to another genetics appointment today. Another stab at this topic, to see if there is anything I can do – and at this stage there is nothing, apart from not get pregnant. As I am taking tamoxifen, it is vital that I do not become pregnant – now that I am on this rollercoaster for five years I must just wait. The risk I am taking is that tamoxifen can bring on the menopause, and if it does – well, that is just life. If it does not then we can revisit that area of harvesting eggs, but for the moment it is a hospital-free world.

This is something that I know I must accept but I am devastated. I don't want to miss the chance to have children of my own but I simply have no choice if I do not want to put myself at risk. I am sure I will learn to accept this news, but not today.

Thursday 25 October

HURRAY! Something amazing happened today. Something good. Thank you the British Government!

Since the beginning of this fiasco I have been entitled to NOTHING! I am a freelance skipper and therefore am entitled to no financial help at all – no reductions, no grants, no sick leave or cover – nothing has been given free. I will never understand why.

Despite paying my taxes and my National Insurance I am advised that because I am freelance I have no rights and no support. That is the risk one takes, apparently, when one leaves the safety of a company. Because I have savings then I can support myself.

I must tell you, however, that the only reason I have some money in the bank is because I sorted myself out immediately I was diagnosed to prepare myself for the onslaught of monthly bills and extra medical fees, drugs and hospital visits and no way of paying them if I was unable to work.

This is a battle I will continue to fight – man alive if I can battle breast cancer I can certainly battle the forces that have done their utmost to provide as little assistance as possible. I will be back.

However, whilst it is a far cry from helping with my utilities, fuel and food, today I received a reduction in my gym fees, to 'help me get back into health'. Oh they won't help me with treatment, diagnosis and the breast cancer nightmare at the time but they will, if you survive, give you a leg up!

Charming!

Mind you, as I don't like to look a gift horse in the mouth I strolled into my local gym armed with my special Healthworks prescription ready to run for my life.

Thursday 8 November

It is one year since the news of my diagnosis rocketed through me and my family and I am still here! I am preparing to head out to the Canaries to return to the start line of that transatlantic yacht race. I promised myself I would be there, and I think I might just make it.

I have spent much of today thinking about last year, remembering that dreadful car journey home from the airport with my parents. This brought on more tears, as I think it will for some time. Thankfully Rich was around today to deal with me.

Saturday 10 November

Almost one year has gone by since we made a tremendously optimistic and perhaps foolhardy commitment to one another as a family that we would raise a glass to a healthy future. Well here we are and we have kept that promise to one another and have spent today at my parents' home, sipping champagne, surrounded by my family, toasting my success at beating my blowfish! This is just fantastic! I think we all deserve this.

I appreciate that it is not that simple – but for now, today, it is!

Wednesday 14 November

A monumental day for me, full of anxiety however, as this morning I left England for Gran Canaria, one of the Canary Islands, to return to the start line of that transatlantic yacht race that I was to skipper a year ago. The race that got away – until now!

I arrived at the dockside and was met by my first mate, Tim, and we clambered about our boat, named, rather unusually, *EH01*. I am one boob lighter but I am more determined than ever to cross that start line in a little over a week.

Tim and I spent much of the day talking, and we began to prepare our boat for the race, bound for St Lucia.

Thursday 15 November

One year ago today I was wheeled into the operating theatre for my mastectomy and embarked on what would turn out to be a rollercoaster of a ride full of fears, highs and lows, laughter and many, many tears.

I awoke in my cabin. I was in a small, hot bunk on my boat in Las Palmas but was absolutely delighted to be here. There was nowhere else in the world I wanted to be this morning. I thought back to what I was doing this time a year ago and chose not to dwell on it. It seemed, for now at least, a million miles away.

Sunday 18 November

Our transatlantic race crew arrived this afternoon, and after some very brief introductions we headed out to meet with Rich and his business partner. There are two boats entering this race for Rich's company, Global Yacht Racing, out of a fleet of well over two hundred, and both myself and the other skipper, Finn, were formally introduced to our crews this evening. A successful evening followed as we began to get to know one another – after all we will be living in extremely close quarters for the next three weeks.

Monday 19 November

I said my goodbyes to Rich and he returned to the UK for a short time before heading down to Sydney. I shall see him again in three weeks' time when I fly into Sydney to meet his family and to co-skipper the Sydney to Hobart yacht race with him.

And so to work. This yacht race is, for many, a once-in-a-life-time challenge. The Atlantic Rally for Cruisers (ARC) is a well-known transatlantic yacht race which began some years ago and has since become a tried and tested route for sailors wishing to embark on a safe, fun, yet challenging transatlantic passage.

Under the watchful eyes of both Tim and myself, our novice crew will leave the Canaries on board our trusted steed *EH01*, after only one week's training, together with the other two hundred and thirty-five yachts, and take on Mother Nature and her ocean and all she has to offer.

I held a meeting with everyone on board this morning, to reintroduce myself and Tim, to provide an opportunity for them to ask any questions that they may have regarding this challenge of a lifetime, to reassure them of our commitment to their challenge and to highlight the experience we have in offshore racing.

I have drawn up a list of tasks for us as a team to complete before departure in under one week – to include training the crew. I have scheduled a training session out on the water each day during both daylight and night-time hours. Sailing at night is very different from sailing during the day as the loss of one of the senses – sight – makes life incredibly difficult. With safety of paramount importance we trained with lifejackets and harnesses on, which restricted their ability to move but was highly amusing to watch from the helm! Sailing is not a glamorous or graceful sport.

Wednesday 21 November

With the contents of our food lockers laid out on the pontoon, some of the crew down below weighing out Skittles, raisins and peanuts in little goodie bags for each crew member and the remainder of the team dividing the boil-in-the-bag meals into sections we created the day bags in sufficient number to cover the length of the race, to include emergency food for another five days at sea.

We only have one food fidget with dietary issues on board. My mate, Tim, is wheat-intolerant and has quickly acquired the fond nickname of 'Special Needs'. This means that he will be unable to eat the boil-in-the-bag meals that the rest of the crew will be enjoying. A cupboard was allotted for his food and instructions were given for his menu to be created. Special Needs was catered for!

I found this name very amusing but I am not sure why I am laughing – the crew nicknamed me 'Cruella', as in Cruella de Vil! Charming!

Bottles of water were brought on board and stowed in vast quantities under every floor board. We do not have a water-maker on board so I shall be rationing the crew to four litres of water a day – which, in the temperatures we shall be experiencing, is barely sufficient.

Friday 23 November

I took Tim for an early drink this evening as I had something to celebrate. Today my periods started again, which was fabulous – although rubbish timing, as I was about to embark on a trans-atlantic yacht race. But nevertheless they had returned and I was so excited. This one tiny thing made such a potential difference to my future and I wanted to tell the world – but in the absence of Rich it was poor Tim that I turned to. Part of his role as my mate, I wonder?

We both admitted that this was not something we would normally celebrate, but he could see the joy in my face and fully understood the implications of this moment for me.

Delightfully, and with much more excitement, we were joined by the whole crew, and together we celebrated Tim's engagement to the lovely Liz, an Irish girl with the softest Irish accent I have ever heard, a girl I have got to know during the race preparations. She is racing too, but on a different boat. The love birds will be reunited in St Lucia.

Saturday 24 November

After first despatching my one female crew member to the laundry I asked my remaining all-male crew if they had all finished with my red nail varnish. Now I know you all now have a vision of seventy little red-painted toes drying in the sun in preparation for their two-week suntan holiday but I am afraid I am going to have to disillusion you – the nail varnish was for their head torches. Far more practical!

I took five minutes today to take stock of where we are. The *EH01* transatlantic race campaign began in anger one week ago. My crew arrived fresh-faced in Las Palmas ready for the adventure of a lifetime. Seven eager beavers and my invaluable first mate Tim – all bright and sparkly – have sat patiently through interminable safety briefs and boat-handling instructions, and to their credit they didn't wiggle once. Their reward? An alarm call at 0630 every morning to begin a frenetic day of boat and crew preparations, together with sailing practice. After all, we've only had seven days to create a race-ready boat and team. From day one I have been in no doubt that we would achieve this but we have needed to put in the hours.

The crew have worked admirably during this preparation week and our little boat, which is to take us all safely from the wilds of windy Gran Canaria to the warm tropical climates of St Lucia, has been scrubbed to within an inch of her life. She has undergone full rig check and sail checks and continues her maintenance programme. She has been loaded to the gunwales with water, diesel and provisions for our adventure.

Sunday 25 November

Race day has dawned and my emotions are running high. This was the race that nearly got away! A little over one year ago, when I was about to skipper this boat from Gibraltar to the start line of this race I received a call that was to change my life forever. I was feeling hugely emotional, and in an effort to hold back the tears I wandered up to the bow for a moment with myself on the pretence of checking that the lines were set properly. I don't think I fooled Special Needs, who joined me on the bow just to see if I was alright.

We slipped lines and headed out of the marina. The noise from the horns, the bands and the cheering was wonderful, and judging by the little faces of my crew they were soaking it all up. A race start is a truly wonderful experience – and for me this one held a particularly special place in my heart too.

We rounded the marina entrance, through the start gate and motored off to examine the start line. Two hundred and thirty-five boats were milling around in the outer harbour area of Las Palmas together with the committee vessel, which was a huge warship. Fortunately the container port had been closed for the race start so there was no commercial shipping movement to contend with at this time. We settled into our race-day start positions and hoisted the mainsail and genoa and tacked and gybed our way around the mayhem waiting patiently for our ten, five and one-minute signals. Finally, with a fantastic boom from the cannon, we crossed the line. Next stop St Lucia.

It was a fast and frantic hour before the race start out on the water, but once over the line a calm fell over the crew as we focused just a little on what we were all about to undertake. This is a familiar body of water for me but for everyone else on board it was a first ocean crossing. Our team song blasted out from the deck speakers and I watched the faces of my crew, with grins from ear to ear, taking in the atmosphere.

One happy skipper!

As the afternoon rolled on into night we began our watch systems with my watch – the Gin Watch – taking the first turn at the helm. Tonic Watch was sent to bed for a snooze with promises to be woken at 2300 hours. A fairly hairy night followed, with the winds, which had been fast and furious all day, not letting up. We had been given a beautiful downwind start with wind speeds of twenty-five to thirty knots gusting upwards but with a heavy sea which was challenging for the helm. We sailed out south-easterly just on the outside edge of the acceleration zone that sits at the south-eastern end of the island. We then turned early evening in the general direction of St Lucia, content in the knowledge that we had gone far enough to clear the dead zone that sits fifty to sixty miles off the southern limits of the island itself. Not so. At around 0300 hours this morning our winds dropped from a fabulous thirty knots to a rather depressing eight knots in the space of about two minutes and so we sat gently moving forwards desperately seeking the wind. We changed the sail pattern accordingly and waited. It was a comfort to learn that we were not alone in our wind hole, as the many navigation lights that surrounded us signalled the predicament of other competitors too.

The crew, now all fed and watered, are still talking to one another so all is well on board. The boat is beginning to smell delightful and the bug that has been raging through the boat and team for the past five days on shore appears to be subsiding.

Monday 26 November

Day two on the Big Brother Boat and no-one has been evicted – all nine of us remain on board and all nine of us in high spirits.

The crew have settled in, with various routines kicking into gear. The teamwork is great with nothing too much trouble. In the lighter airs of this afternoon a punishing schedule of sail changes and goose-winging, topped with me promptly changing my mind (thanks to Mother Nature's indecisiveness!), had both

Gin and Tonic Watches on their toes seeking every gust of wind. Our efforts were rewarded with a spirit-lifting sail past three of our competitors.

Earlier this afternoon we spotted a yacht heading in our direction with a large black mainsail and no headsail up. Curiously we watched as she crossed our path in the direction of Africa. As she drew nearer we spotted the unmistakable logo of *Pi Squared*, our Global Yacht Racing competition. This unusual course and sail configuration sparked concerns of an injury on board, so I attempted to make contact on the VHF. With an eerie silence I resorted to an email. I was later to discover that the crew had decided on race start day to pop vast amounts of seasickness tablets in anticipation of a breezy day, which promptly sent them all to sleep. Finn and his mate were left to sail the long and heavy night alone. Still, all well in the end – but encouraging for the troops on board *EH01* as we were at least heading in the right direction.

Once again the fashion of the ever-so-sexy sport of ocean yacht racing never ceases to amaze me. We are now at that crucially confusing phase of temperatures that are warming up but are not quite there yet to allow us to shed all the layers, so the traditional combination of shorts over thermal bottoms with T-shirt, hat, jacket, sun glasses and head torch returns with the arrival of Gin Watch on deck. My crew are feeling somewhat self-conscious about their image. This will soon change.

Tonight brought the first taste for many on board of the boil-in-the-bag experience. A crucial one in ocean racing! The chosen menu for today was delicious spicy meatballs with pasta for lunch followed by Lancashire hotpot for supper – all served in the traditional and elegant foil bag heated in fresh sea water. I think perhaps I have been ocean racing too long, as I actually love these meals. The crew have yet to be convinced, judging by the looks on their faces. My theory is always begin with the best to lull them into a false sense of security and then bring in the big guns. The chicken performance is revolting so I have arranged that for day seven. (Well, I am led to believe that is what lurks at the bottom of the foil bag marked 'chicken casserole', but I have been looking for some years now and have yet to discover the truth!)

Unfortunately the wind has dropped a little this evening with a resultant drop in our speed but with the good winds scheduled for return early dawn tomorrow we remain buoyant.

With a chorus of 'You are my sunshine' Gin Watch settled in to their remaining three hours whilst their team-mates slept.

Wednesday 28 November

Day four and a subdued crew stumble erratically onto deck. Those that have made it through the returning stomach bug are fragile and sit curled up in the cockpit – a banana clutched in a hot little hand is the chosen food for this stage in their recovery. Those that are still sick remain curled up in their bunks and Tim and I run between whatever we can to cover the hours, sleeping fully clothed in foulies and lifejackets on the spinnakers down below when necessary. Fortunately those that are up are great drivers, allowing us a little rest time. Thankfully though there are two more faces up and about today than there were yesterday – I think we are now just one man down.

With the wind direction as it was this morning I decided we were being pushed too far north so we popped in a gybe and turned south. Needless to say, as we had just settled ourselves in the wind sped up and backed, this time pushing us too far around, so we gybed back and poled out the headsail, allowing us to make a direct beeline for the finish.

The afternoon ticked by quite uneventfully, the odd dolphin but not much to speak of – but, following a brief star constellation lecture a few nights ago, the now regular nightly search for Cassiopeia's Chair began in earnest this evening, followed by Orion and his belt and the Great Bear and Polaris. The starry nights are quite definitely the highlight of any ocean passage with no light pollution at all, and to date they have not disappointed – they are absolutely amazing.

One of the highlights of this transatlantic yacht race is that there are two hundred and thirty odd boats to play with all heading across the Atlantic together, for companionship and safety. The camaraderie out on the water is great. Radio chitchats are often to be heard, and this also means that we get regular updates from race headquarters advising us all of the news, events and dangers too. Sadly we heard this evening of a nasty accident on board a vessel, the injured crew member requiring an evacuation. We also heard of an immigrant situation. Before leaving Las Palmas, at the skippers' briefing, we were advised of the problem of immigrant boats that set off from Africa, one hundred or so people crammed into long low boats for up to five days at a time. They are trying to get to the first available land, in this case the Canary Islands. Apparently if these long boats spot a yacht they make a beeline for it and attempt to board. We were advised what we should do under these circumstances. And this evening we have learned that a yacht in the race has been boarded by two immigrants who have been restrained by the crew. The situation is now in the hands of the authorities. It is a busy piece of water out here!

Personally, I have been expecting the normal nightly bombardment by the flying fish brigade that litter an ocean passage, but nothing as yet. Very disappointing. We are five days into an ocean passage and we still haven't been hit in the face by a wet fish. All that is still to come!

Friday 30 November

Good progress.

The Boil-in-the-bag Olympics got under way this morning with a full complement of crew in action once again. The events started with the Dumpling Long Shot. A rather unwelcome addition to the beef stew, the dumpling had to be launched by use of the spoon held in the left hand only over the left shoulder upwind – making each competitor aware of his or her surroundings and bringing an extra dynamic to the sport. This tests the wind awareness of the yacht race competitors.

Tonic Watch (aka maintenance crew) continued their daily routine of discovering new items to mend during the night watch. (I might point out that if they didn't keep breaking things then they wouldn't have to mend them!) Since the excitement earlier in the week of the broken vang we have only experienced a couple of maintenance issues. A mainsail slider has failed and some attention is needed on the steering cable, otherwise our floating home is serving us well.

I think we may have finally beaten the bug! After two deep cleans using bleach and anti-bac and a further deep clean today, all crew are now on their feet and eating. I am keeping my fingers crossed. Thankfully all the team have found their sea legs, and in fact seasickness has not been an issue for anyone in the team to date.

Tim 'Special Needs' continues to torment his watch with his cooking prowess, producing tasty meals for himself from fresh food and non-wheat products. Although the Wayfarer food has proved to be better than expected, the menu is now starting to repeat itself. Tim's daily dishes, on the other hand, seem to be new and different flavoured concoctions each day.

———

Holy Moly! What an episode!

The past two hours have been challenging to say the least. Six hours ago, I awoke to a tremendous corkscrewing feeling, the feeling of a boat not quite in its groove. The sea state was making our progress on our intended track untenable so I made the decision to put in a gybe and a reef some twenty-four hours earlier than I would have liked. We settled the boat down again and I went back to bed. Tonic Watch continued until the 2300 hours watch change.

So, with Tonic Watch safely tucked into their bunks, Gin Watch began their four-hour 'graveyard' shift with quiet stargazing once again – and then ... wallop! Mother Nature did her bit again and took the wind from 15 knots to 30 knots in a second, knocking us flat and requiring some immediate action. We dropped the headsail and changed it for a slightly smaller hand-kerchief-sized one and reefed the mainsail for more control. The sea swell was also still doing its level best to make life as uncomfortable as possible. Once the boat was under control I took the helm and tried, for the remaining two hours of our watch, to persuade the little monkey to behave. She was not having it, though, and fought me every inch of the way. Eventually the sea state subsided a little and the boat speed improved.

Saturday 1 December

It never ceases to amaze me how Mother Nature can be so fickle. After the beating of last night we awake to a much smoother passage. The swell still remains, as does the wind strength, but she has finally decided to play ball with us and the wind has veered around to an east-north-east direction which has allowed us to turn twenty degrees further west – and therefore the swell is not knocking us flat with every wave.

Dawn breaks in the darkness and I realise that we have to move the clocks or we will eventually find ourselves standing in the dark at noon! So today it is then. It stretches each watch by thirty minutes to accommodate the hour but will be better in the long run. The extra time has been used well to clean up below decks, re-stow loose items, flake and pack the number 1 headsail and generally make the boat shipshape again after last night's shenanigans.

I am afraid to say that I spat my dummy early this morning regarding the bilges. And there is a very good reason for this. A friend of ours is currently on a yacht that is heading back to the Cape Verde islands. This is because the yacht was experiencing substantial water ingress via the keel bolts that pass through the hull to hold the keel in place. The ingress cannot be contained and they are frantically bailing to prevent the boat from sinking.

The only way to find out if the keel bolts are leaking is to check under the floors regularly. So I have introduced a column in the log book entitled 'bilge check', which is supposed to ensure that the bilges are being checked on an hourly basis. I note that this column has been ticked hourly but I discovered this afternoon that the floor boards were not being lifted. I admit it is a fiddle to lift the boards as the sails are lying on top of them and need to be moved each time – but nevertheless it is vital that this check is done. To simply tick the box and not do the check is foolhardy, dangerous and unacceptable. A justified dummy spit, I feel!

Other than that a very uneventful day, except we learnt that our direct competition has torn their mainsail. This will hopefully give us an advantage.

The aerial bombardments by squadrons of flying fish are beginning in anger. The little stinky wet fish seem to think it amusing to make night-time stealth raids on our boat. Come daylight, we collect the once desperately flapping little bodies, who had presumably at some point during the night been rolling around the deck clutching their shiny little heads, crying, after hitting either us or the various metal paraphernalia that adorns a deck, and who by the time we gather them up are suffering from severe rigor mortis. If you survive a night without being hit in the face or head by a wet flying fish with a combined head-on velocity of some twenty knots you are doing very well.

Sunday 2 December

Day eight on the Big Brother Boat and tensions flare up over the washing up. Still no-one has been evicted but all boat members were called to the dining room.

Sailing must be the most unflattering sport. Showers are limited or cancelled altogether. It takes at least ten minutes to get all your kit on – and trust me it is exhausting to do at the best of times, let alone when you are being thrown about the boat in big swells.

Well today has been an on/off, up/down day on Gin Watch. On with the foulies, off with the foulies, up with the number 3 headsail, down with the number 3, up goes the number 1 ... You get the picture.

Monday 3 December

We picked up a stalker this morning. There we are, quietly minding our own business, hoofing along at breakfast time, when a yacht crosses our bow from left to right. He then contacts us on the radio for a chitchat. We respond accordingly and he advises us of a broken this, that and the other on his boat. Again we respond accordingly and he advises us that he has access to no weather information. We advise him that we do have access to weather information. He then makes the unusual decision to completely change his course and follow us, and could we advise him when we will be turning to St Lucia! Bless him, he also advises that he 'will keep a safe distance behind us'. This gets my goat a little so I jump on the helm, belt ten miles out of the old girl and now we can only just see his mast! Safe distance, indeed! He can barely see us now.

After a pretty uneventful afternoon, with boat speed and direction all in check, we enjoyed, for the first time, the sun and heat. The rail was littered with crew. It was a great few hours. Tonic Watch kept the boat rocketing along my new heading, which saw us dipping slightly south to avoid a high pressure containing extremely light winds that has plonked itself right in our path for St Lucia.

For the first time in I don't know how many days I just managed to doze off this afternoon when, with great excitement, my mate stumbled into my cabin to advise me that he could see a yacht on the port bow with main down, flapping headsail and an orange emergency sail hanging over the side. We altered course immediately and headed for the stricken vessel, under sail of course as we don't want to bail from the race. I tried to raise them on the radio but to no avail, and as we approached and circled the yacht we took the name from the stern and tried once more. With no response I blasted the fog horn to attract attention, all the while searching the water for a life raft or bodies. Again nothing – and I began to feel uneasy. She was listing, drifting on the swell with the swim ladder down. An inspired thought from one of my crew reminded me of a note that had come through from race headquarters a couple of days earlier speaking of a yacht that had been abandoned. Her crew had been rescued but the yacht would remain drifting. It was clear from the name that we had stumbled across this abandoned yacht. What are the chances of that in such a huge ocean?

It is all go out here today. There has been another abandoned yacht spotted, north and west of us, thankfully, but smelling of fuel. A busy bit of water, this North Atlantic!

Tuesday 4 December

Today dawned with the reality that we still have another 1,500 miles to go and no wind in which to do it. The reality of another fifteen days at sea to achieve this sets in my mind.

The wind hole that we are currently sitting in has not been forecast. Our barometer dropped hourly. We ghosted along this morning with very little wind and chanced a kite – which thankfully held and gave us boat speed of eight knots for a period of about eight hours in a direct line for St Lucia – perfect! A few threatening clouds overhead passed uneventfully, and after four hours of helming I took the opportunity to nip below for a quick snooze.

Silly me – what was I thinking? No sooner was my back turned than the rains finally arrived. The kite was dropped as the squall sat overhead and soaked us. We re-hoisted a headsail to try to keep up boat speed. Sadly, however, our angle was reduced and we returned to being twenty degrees off course. Not such a great course but still a good speed so we could continue to knock off the miles.

During the continued rains I took the opportunity to head to the leeward rail armed with my shampoo for a quick shower. We haven't had showers for ten days and this was too good an opportunity to miss. I was followed by anyone who was up.

A wonderful evening sail with poled-out headsail and the huge sea swell once again ensues. I leave the deck for another attempt at a snooze. Twenty minutes later the sail is back over the other side with the pole down and the mainsail is reefed! The herd of wildebeest that effected this change in sail pattern is now safely grazing in the cockpit once more.

So once more another unpredictable day on the water – and we push on through until dawn.

Wednesday 5 December

Another day on board brings wildlife. With great excitement the crew belted to the bow to watch thirty to forty dolphins close in on the boat. It is truly magical to see them making a beeline for us and then playing with the bow wave, enjoying the speed. These creatures in their natural habitat are amazing.

———

Discussions began in earnest this afternoon as to when we might make land. I gave them my own best estimate of an arrival time, based on the remaining mileage, average speed and potential sailing angles – lit the blue touch paper and retired to watch with amusement the various thought processes undertaken by each crew member to come up with a date and time.

As the evening drew in and dusk settled, the orange hue of the late afternoon disappearing, the now familiar night-time weather pattern approached with waves beginning to build up to ten or twelve feet and the dark clouds rolling in overhead. Clearly it is going to be another uncomfortable night, and it remains to be seen whether we will be able to hold course.

Thursday 6 December

Psssssst! Come closer! I have to whisper this.

Mother Nature messed up today. During one of her wind-free lessons on how to bob around in the middle of the ocean, which she frequently insists we attend, whilst we were going in circles with a little bit of north thrown in (with our destination being just south of west), she slipped up and let out a whole lot of wind which we managed to escape on – and we are now thankfully bound directly for Rodney Bay, St Lucia – the bar in fact – at 8.5 knots.

But don't tell a soul.

We received news from Base Camp Cowes of the position of those yachts in our racing fleet located around us, and after plotting all the other yachts' positions on our chart I discovered that we are currently in sixth place. It is a huge morale boost to see on paper the location of our competitors. Our nearest challenger is thirty miles away and very reachable.

Earlier this evening I pottered down below to do some navigation and perhaps to grab a couple of hours and was awoken by the shaking of the boat as the troops on deck were putting in their second reef. A head popped into my cabin to advise me that we were experiencing thirty knots and could we please change to a smaller headsail. I shot up on deck to see what was happening. The winds had been steadily building to the point where life became pretty uncomfortable and we took fifty knots with higher gusts and seas of twelve to fifteen feet. The boys were sent to the bow to change the sail. As the winds remained at forty-five to fifty knots we also dropped the mainsail and continued under the headsail only, which was much more comfortable and we still kept speed.

Finally – with the winds and seas still raging – Tonic Watch went to bed and Gin Watch started their four-hour vigil to keep the boat safe. A challenging night and one somewhat in contrast to our last week. I checked the weather information I had received and noted that we were due to receive a maximum of ten knots tonight. It just shows that you cannot rely on the weathermen!

Friday 7 December

As dawn broke the crew tentatively lifted their exhausted bodies. The beating of last night clearly evident in their faces, and the carnage strewn both above and below deck, gave it all away. It was a truly sterling effort from them all last night. Watch times were overrun and sleep was at a premium, with very few achieving it. Last night the winds blew and I gave an 'all hands' call – and within minutes the troops were on deck and making our little boat safe.

Our winds dropped to a more manageable thirty to thirty-five knots this morning but the leaden skies remained menacing. The seas were angry and confused with waves still around twelve to fifteen feet. We seemed to spend more time going up and down than going forward so progress was slow. The sea would pick us up on one wave and drop us off at the bottom of a huge trough over and over again, which was heavy and hard work on the body. In my opinion we were spending more time at an unnatural angle than is expected for a downwind race!

We plodded on through the day, and towards the end of the afternoon an unnerving calm took over – the eye-of-a-storm type of calm which makes me very uncomfortable, nervous. I have no means of predicting this particular little gem from Mother Nature. It is still showing ten knots of breeze on the weather files that I download and I am therefore trying to navigate an ocean with no reliable weather information, which makes my job tricky. We rely solely on what we can see and feel throughout this storm, and on our little barometer. I think Mother Nature must be a man!

The crew, encouraged by the strong winds and high boat speeds, have secured their arrival date and time predictions on paper, which are varied and interesting. I have yet to add mine!

During today's squalls some of the crew took it upon themselves to give this free shower business a go and were last seen heading to the leeward rail, their heads already covered in shampoo so as not to waste time once down on the perilous low side.

Saturday 8 December

Woke up on the wall today! I found myself examining the underside of the bunk above me. Needless to say the strong winds that we have been experiencing have not abated and we still battle with reef in, reef out, number 1 down, number 3 up, number 3 down, number 4 up. Exhausting.

The squalls continue to provide the opportunity for showers, and now washing – a bucket was placed in the cockpit for gathering rain water for later use. A few more sail changes followed, after which the full bucket of rain water provided the opportunity to turn the cockpit into a launderette. Socks and underwear were the order of the day and after a fair amount of scrubbing the area was beginning to smell Persil-fresh, with all manner of newly washed items pegged to the rail or wedged under any line that might act as a weight to hold the aforementioned smalls down in the breeze.

Less than one hour after the final squall, for us on Gin Watch, the tides appeared to have turned – the sun shone, the wind dropped to a very pleasant twenty knots, the reefs came out, the headsails were made bigger to capitalise on the wonderful new flat sea state and I sat – nervous of what was around the corner. Just as the storm had come in without warning it appeared to have left the same way. I remained unconvinced

The fleet appears to have suffered enormously with this storm, with dismastings, broken booms, hull damage, abandonments and evacuations. The list was endless – and all because this storm was not predicted and people were unprepared for what lay in wait for them. It is carnage out here.

It is the little things you take for granted, I noted during a particularly challenging dressing episode this morning – such as a horizontal bedroom floor and the ability to get dressed without holding onto the bedroom wall, or going to the bathroom without lurching for the door frame.

Sunday 9 December

A rather uneventful and calm evening with winds decreasing rapidly to frustration levels of two knots coming from the west resulted in us pirouetting for some time – and then it picked up again and turned everything into another bun fight. We were once again overpowered and had an 'all hands' call to reduce and peel the foresails. Once again you will not be surprised to learn that this storm was not predicted on the weather files, just another ten knots downwind.

We are trucking along through the remaining five hundred odd miles, edging our way closer to St Lucia. Talk of hotel rooms and hot baths is rearing its ugly head, which is a sure-fire way to jinx us. The squalls continue to come in, soaking all on deck, but I guess at least it is warm and you can dry out during the sunny spells.

Monday 10 December

We have had a chilled-out cultural day today on board. Finally we have been able to bask in the sunshine that is well overdue for this race, and with a boat speed of nine knots all day set against a backdrop of beautiful warm trade winds we have, as a crew, enjoyed a sewing circle repairing the sails, some chilled music and an 'under five hundred miles' treat made by Special Needs – a fruit crumble.

If this continues I think we shall be in for breakfast on Thursday.

Tomorrow is shower day. At the outset I promised the crew that if we had enough water two days out from St Lucia we could all have a shower so, true to my word, tomorrow is shower day. This is handy, as we all smell horrible. We have been bathing in baby wet wipes and some of us have managed to have a rain hair wash, which was heaven. The water for these showers will be monitored and the pump will be controlled from the navigation desk.

We paid dearly for our chilled-out afternoon with an arse kicking tonight. It began in earnest just after supper and continued long into the early hours. I broke my watch this evening and they are off to bed for a couple of hours to recharge their batteries.

Tuesday 11 December

Dawn broke over the horizon this morning. No beautiful sunrise of red and gold, just rain clouds, dark and foreboding.

Mother Nature did her worst again last night. She clearly

intends to make us work every inch of this race course. She is relentless and exhausting. I bet as we cross the line into the beautiful Rodney Bay she will be blowing a hooley!

We were given a treat this morning, though, in exchange for our troubles last night. Dolphins! Three: mummy, daddy and a tiny baby. All three leaping so high – I have crossed this ocean more times than I care to think about and never seen dolphins leap so high, they were amazing. This was topped off by a beautiful and bright rainbow which arced over us set against a black cloudy sky that only served to accentuate its beauty. We seemed to sail right underneath it. She had a shadow too which mimicked her own crisp shape with both ends clearly visible. What a lovely start!

We discovered this morning that we are still powering ahead of our direct competitor, the other Global Yacht Racing boat, *Pi Squared*, by a healthy margin of one hundred and fifty miles – which is fantastic news and a great morale boost in these horrible conditions.

We are now on the final Food Day Bag, and between us we have managed to pick our way through the Wayfarers, eating as much as we all wanted – but we are now left with a selection of spotted dick, sausage casserole, Skittles and peanuts in their hundreds and a rather dodgy Spanish Mars Bar type affair which has not been popular. My father makes a fantastic sausage casserole, and when I first discovered that we had a boil-in-the-bag version I waited excitedly for the day when this would be pulled from the Day Bag. Disappointment followed. The 'sausages' were like rubber bullets, pale and uninteresting, but they bounced very well – they make tinned frankfurters look appetising!

I did some navigation homework and noted that to date we have sailed 2,900 miles from Las Palmas, and I believe we have around two hundred to go until we reach those well-earned cool beers. We rocketed through a lovely 195 miles in the last twenty-four hours, which is pleasing.

As the first night watch settled in after a scorching afternoon the wind picked up once again. We are fortunate now in that we have been able to make a beeline directly for the northern end of St Lucia, having spent the past ten hours heading a little north of our preferred course due to wind angle. The sea state is huge and comes at us broadside. I must admit in the dark I am finding it terribly difficult to judge it. The crew have been phenomenal on the helm throughout.

Thursday 13 December

Guess what. We are still out here. Very frustrating.

Friday 14 December

I was right! As we rounded Pigeon Island at the northern tip of St Lucia bound for Rodney Bay Mother Nature did her worst and just as I predicted she blew. Unperturbed, and with our team song blaring out from the deck speakers, we tacked our way across the finish line. Cheers roared out from both the crew and the committee vessel which marked one end of the finish line and whose fog horn signalled our finish and registered our finish time. I looked around the deck at my crew, who were delighted and very proud of themselves.

What an amazing experience. I was tingling all over and sported a grin from ear to ear! I had just kept the promise I made to myself in the summer of 2006 and skippered my first ocean race, and it was a truly fabulous experience, made even more special by the cancer false start of last year.

The daytime finish was perfect. The crew packed away the deck and the sails were dropped. Lines and fenders made their first appearance on deck in nearly three weeks. We motored into the marina and received rapturous applause from those yacht crews who were already in. I reversed *EHo1* into our given berth, where we were met by friends and family – and a journalist.

Wasting just the one bottle of champagne over my head, the

crew and I began the celebrations. I thanked my crew for their team work, camaraderie, herculean effort, humour and sheer determination to make this transatlantic yacht race a success. I advised them of our fourth place listing and took another sip of bubbles.

The rest of the day has been a bit of a blur.

Saturday 15 December

The journalist returned this morning to do an interview with me regarding the boat we found bobbing around out in the deep earlier this month.

Reluctantly the crew rose to the challenge of returning *EH01* to a healthy and happy state. She reeked! Nearly three weeks at sea, nine dirty bodies, filthy clothes, stinky wet shoes and a sickness bug have all taken their toll on the poor old girl. After first removing all the rubbish, sails, stores and personal kit they cleaned *EH01* to within an inch of her life once more.

Sunday 16 December

Today is departure day. I am off to Australia. Me, my prosthesis and I. She still has no name, but that doesn't stop her being in preparation for her third international yacht race. Her log book is looking quite healthy with the Fastnet and the ARC, her first transatlantic, already tucked under her belt this year. The Sydney to Hobart is the next race in her sights. I wonder how far south a prosthesis has travelled.

She and I have come to rely on one another over the past months. Me for her help in making me look a little less like a lopsided freak and a little more balanced, and she on me for her exciting lifestyle and international travels. She should be pleased. One slight hand movement from the nurse who gave me my prosthesis all those months ago might have resulted in picking up the box next to hers, and she could have been sad-dled with domestic normality: attached to the chest of a woman doing normal stuff, the school run, dropping little Isabella and Toby at the Montessori in Upper West-Wotsit! Instead she sails the oceans of the globe, which I hope she finds much more fun!

I wonder if there is a weight advantage to sailing with only one boob.

My first hurdle, however, is a long-overdue meeting with Rich's huge family.

Tuesday 18 December

Finally I arrived in Sydney. One year late.

It is not exactly a direct flight from St Lucia to Sydney. I had to fly first to Puerto Rico, then on to Los Angeles, where I had an eight-hour wait before boarding my final flight to Sydney. With my fear of flying really kicking in these days I found this journey very unpleasant, although I did manage to catch up on about three weeks' sleep – knowing that I was no longer responsible for nine lives and a yacht.

I was met by Rich, who arrived in Sydney a few days ago and was in full swing with the preparations for the Sydney to Hobart race, which leaves on Boxing Day. Just a week to go and still so much to do.

However, it was wonderful to see him and to finally make it down to Australia. He was very excited to show me around, introduce me to his friends and family and generally show me his home.

Monday 24 December

We drove up to the Blue Mountains today to join some of Rich's family for Christmas, briefly. Sadly we will have to leave late on Christmas Day to return to Sydney for pre-race skipper and weather briefings. However, the break was wonderful.

I was very nervous. I have met one sister and one niece – but with a further four sisters, two brothers, two sisters-in-law, four brothers-in-law, seven nieces, three nephews and an aunt still to go I am going to be in trouble with names! To my knowledge I will be meeting all of them this visit, to include the sister and brother-in-law in Hobart when we get there. The one sister in Mexico might just escape the visit this time.

I needn't have worried. I was welcomed with open arms by the whole family, nineteen members at this count. Rich has two sisters who live up near the mountains and we began at one house and moved, en masse, to the next.

Rich pulled an ace card today – he introduced me, and then as his family began to surround me he backed away and grabbed a cold beer with one of his brothers and watched. As I disappeared under hugs and kisses I felt very welcome and very happy – what a fantastic family. I think I am going to like being a Falk.

The afternoon and evening became a warm and happy affair with plenty of food and wine, stories of a young Rich – a true family event surrounded by loved ones. I was most definitely being welcomed into the bosom of a large warm and loving family.

I am the girl that their little brother is to marry, and they have had to wait one year to meet me! I hope I lived up to their expectations today. Personally, I had a wonderful day. I looked over to Rich lying next to me and wondered what he was thinking. I hope he enjoyed himself.

Wednesday 26 December

Race day today. The atmosphere on the pontoons was electric. It was hot and sunny and the skippers were putting their crews through the final team briefings. There was noise and chaos everywhere, sails and various other nautical paraphernalia adorned the pontoons, and there were the familiar sights and sounds of pre-race preparations tinged with an element of last-minute panic. This is an annual highlight for the city, and the public interest is always enormous.

The Sydney to Hobart is Australia's most famous offshore race. It is a truly challenging six-hundred-and-twenty-mile race lasting anything between thirty-six hours and six days, depending on your boat. The course takes the fleet out through Sydney Heads, down the east coast of Australia bound for Tasmania, across the Bass Strait and dipping a toe in the top of the Southern Ocean. The fleet sails through several weather systems with a guaranteed pasting from a deep low-pressure system on the approach to Tasmania. This iconic event is one that offshore sailors from all over the world aspire to compete in – a Holy Grail in offshore racing.

The press were everywhere, and once again their interest in me was sweet – an ordinary girl with an inspirational story of achievement. A 'feel-good factor story', they called me. I found myself in the papers once again – which was weird but exciting, flattering.

Sydney Harbour was buzzing. Support vessels of all shapes and sizes crammed into the pre-race area along with the race yachts, making our exit towards the start line chaotic.

The Sydney to Hobart yacht race is attracts many sailors from the Northern Hemisphere, and as we crossed the start line I found myself thinking – another tick in a box of things I want to achieve.

Friday 28 December

Two days into the race.

I began experiencing some discomfort, a sharp pain, around my lower stomach. I chose to ignore it for the moment as there was nothing that could be done, I was at sea, and frankly it was not stopping me from doing anything. I was still able to run around, hoist sails and generally perform my role as co-skipper. So with great determination we continued south to Hobart.

This race is known for its volatile waters. Nine years ago, in 1998, an intense low-pressure system swept through the race fleet whipping up monstrous seas with its high winds. Five boats sank, six people died, and only forty-four of the one hundred and fifteen starters made it to Hobart – with one of the smallest yachts, skippered by a friend of ours, crossing the finishing line in first place.

Sunday 30 December

We crossed the finish line early this afternoon. I have finished my first Sydney to Hobart Yacht Race. An electric finish once again, with a carnival atmosphere on the pontoons. As Rich parked the boat in our berth I heard my name. I was met by a smiling face and was introduced to another sister-in-law to be. Penny and her husband John had come down to see our arrival, which was wonderful for us both. With a particularly busy time still ahead of us as always at the end of a race we arranged to go and spend some time with them in a couple of days, when we could relax and enjoy more family hospitality.

Tuesday 1 January 2008

A simple trip to the nearest brasserie in the centre of Hobart to collect a much-needed bacon and egg butty for one slightly hungover husband-to-be turned into a media event.

I stood quietly in line with two other members of our race crew who had, it appeared, beaten the bacon butty rush by already placing their orders. As I was intermittently reading the front page of the New Year's Day papers and chatting with my crew I noted a bit of pointing and whispering rippling around the room. My crew noticed this too and suggested that I turn the paper over to read the sports page, and in particular the sailing section. Staring back at me was a grinning picture of – well, me! A large photograph and full-page story on this 'brave cancer survivor', under the headline 'Emma's dying wish'. Oh my God! I was splashed all over the back pages!

After the media attention I received in Sydney on my arrival I thought all had calmed a little, but it appeared that the interest in me had travelled south with the race fleet. The media's continued belief in me and my drive to go on living life – and such an energetic one, having only cleared breast cancer barely two months previously – was the feel-good story that they all wanted. This in itself is terribly flattering for me, and it makes me feel even more determined.

Once again, the article is wonderful, but it makes it sound as if I am dying of cancer, as if I have failed in my efforts to beat my blowfish – and the whole thing knocked me a little. I don't remember speaking to this journalist, but I have spoken to a number by now. I am particularly shocked by the headline.

Thursday 3 January

Remaining in severe discomfort and unhappy about setting sail whilst suffering from the same pains I had experienced during the race, I checked myself into the accident and emergency department of the private, and ridiculously expensive, Hobart Hospital – where I proceeded to sit and wait for four hours with the long-suffering Erica wasting her final day in Hobart at my side.

Eventually I was seen by a South African doctor who, on discovering my Cornish roots, announced that he had spent time practising on the Isles of Scilly during my father's years there as the Land Steward.

I tried to explain my feelings, and brought to his attention my experience with breast cancer. It was not a successful consultation, and I made a note to discuss my situation with Rich's brother Paul, who is a doctor. His assistance and advice have been fabulous, and I will be forever grateful. Actually I have been so very lucky having so many medical experts in the family to turn to – not only Paul but also Trish, who is a nurse, and Ranna, a radiographer – all bases covered, and all have played a huge role in calming me down and supporting both Rich and me in a very relaxed fashion – which for someone like me is vital.

Monday 14 January

Back in Sydney, I remain displeased with my consultation in the very expensive and very exclusive hospital in Hobart, from where I had been sent packing clutching a prescription for omeprazole, a drug I have become very familiar with over the past year which is prescribed to cancer patients undergoing chemotherapy.

I had been particularly anxious this morning as I underwent a PET scan. Positron emission tomography. The more familiar CT and MRI scans are not able to detect active tumours, whereas a PET scan measures the body's abnormal molecular activity and creates a picture of how my body's cells are functioning. It is designed to spot actively growing cancerous cells. It can apparently pick them up when they are the size of a grain of rice. Amazing!

I am afraid that this is all part of my cancerphobia – the need to be scanned and checked to keep an eye on me. I am finding it difficult to move on. I have been terrified that something has been missed, so I arranged to undergo this scan.

After first injecting a type of dye, a radioactive glucose, into my bloodstream the nurses left me to sit quietly for one hour, following which I was scanned from top to toe. Not a particularly unpleasant experience, the PET scan is simple, painless and fast (and just a little bit nerve-wracking), but something that, if results are all clear, will give me a feeling of closure. There was no stone that would be left unturned.

We returned home to wait. A particularly uncomfortable

time. I was fidgety and nervous, but by early afternoon we had received a call to say that all was well and that the only cause for concern was that the scan had picked up a couple of cysts on the ovaries – which were of no particular concern as they are a common symptom in women taking tamoxifen.

So I was diagnosed as having ovarian cysts, which would explain the pain and discomfort I had been experiencing during the race. And yet the doctor in Hobart had put it all down to stress after my breast cancer. Surely a simple ultrasound would have revealed the truth?

Friday 25 January

Time for contemplation this evening. It is one year since I was given my first dose of chemotherapy, and I had many months of treatment still ahead of me. I am now able to look back at that time with relief and encouragement. However, I regularly have moments of self-pity, which I guess is to be expected.

I have been humbled incredibly during my visit to Australia. Whilst Rich and I were there I was introduced to some of his friends, one of whom, Tony, is blind and carries a stick. Tony is truly an amazing man. He has nine lives, of that I am sure. A fit and active person, a talented sailor and pilot, Tony has survived a plane crash from which he and his family walked away. He has been resuscitated after his heart stopped shortly after completing a yacht race. He survived the carnage of the infamous 1998 Sydney to Hobart yacht race but had his legs crushed – and the reason this man stood before me with a white stick in his hand was because he and his wife were caught in the recent bombing of Bali, in which he was badly injured and lost his sight.

Tony returned to Tasmania after our Sydney to Hobart race. He had flown down to join some friends who were delivering their race yacht back to Sydney, for even without sight Tony's feel for the motion of the water gives him an amazing ability to helm, and he derives a huge amount of enjoyment from being out on the water with his friends.

A cheeky character with so much life inside him. When I first met him I felt something on my leg when I was standing talking to him and looked down to discover Tony moving his stick up my leg. He turned to Rich and retorted, 'I'm just having a look!'

I looked again at this incredible man, who sported a grin from ear to ear and who was enjoying a beer with his friends. Life was clearly not going to get him down and I felt any remnants of self-pity leave and my determination and stubbornness build – he gave me great strength to fight, whatever the situation. For me, he was truly amazing.

Tuesday 29 January

We went on our second visit to see Mr Whitworth, my reconstruction surgeon, who would confirm and explain in further detail the surgery I was to undergo. We talked at length, and it was decided that I should remain on the list for a right prophylactic mastectomy and full reconstruction. I was delighted. This would signal the end of this nightmare for me. Fully reconstructed and looking like a normal girl again – and with my own hair – I could get married!

Wednesday 30 January

Today we went to the first of a series of three-monthly checkups to see my oncologist and to report in. These checkups will be a regular part of my life for the next five years. I was very nervous, which is to be expected I guess, but the lovely thing about these longer gaps in between seeing Peter is that there is enough time for me to forget what I have been through just a little. It gives me a break from it all – and then suddenly I am brought back to earth with a bump. Back to the hospital appointments, to the room where it all began.

Fortunately today was a good day, and Peter sent me away with a grin on my face. There was nothing of any concern that he had picked up, and I had nothing to report to him. I did of course take with me the details of the PET scan I underwent in Australia and mentioned the results which showed the ovarian cysts. I confirmed that I was not experiencing the pains I had previously felt, but exercising caution he organised an ultrasound scan just to check on these cysts.

Tuesday 5 February

Had a shot with my hairdryer and brush today, with disastrous results. I don't think I am quite at that stage yet. My hair is definitely growing at a great rate but the need for outside implements is not here yet.

Sunday 10 February

With all my savings used up paying bills that I must meet, but without a reliable source of regular income, my finances are becoming an issue. Some people are still very nervous about employing me, concerned that I am not up to the job. This is ridiculous if you consider my track record – which has even been publicly written about in numerous national and international papers.

I have been able to continue to sail throughout my treatment, and I have even been able to skipper a transatlantic yacht race and the Sydney to Hobart. However, some people just will not believe.

I learnt only recently that if I were to de-register as a freelance and register as unemployed and receive a jobseeker's allowance I could receive £19,000 per annum – now how does that work?

Wednesday 13 February

In four weeks time I shall undergo my right prophylactic mastectomy together with a full reconstruction and silicone breast implants.

That was the news I received today, and although elated – as this is what Rich and I have been waiting for – I was subdued. It will feel like I am returning to the start of this nightmare, returning to hospital again to undergo another unpleasant operation, another mastectomy, another period with restrictive drains sewn into my chest, another week of relying solely on other people to get by, to wash, to cook, to reach out and live life normally, and then a further few weeks of regaining movement in my arms and feeling in my chest. Do I really want to put myself through this? With the mastectomy there was no choice – well, not if I wanted to live – but this is pure vanity. To have two boobs is not a lot to ask, but I will be returning to the start. All the hard work I have put in over the last year, getting back on top, sailing, skippering and returning to my independence, will seem wasted. I have played with this thought all day and will continue to do so, I am sure.

I call my girlfriends and report the news – 'Pammy (*as in Pamela Anderson*) is on her way' – and they are delighted, excited and, oddly, a little envious. Not a word I would associate with me and my experiences over the past year but nevertheless a word that was used.

You see, to me, the decision to remove the right breast is simple. I have no intention of returning to chemotherapy and radiotherapy. Both are very useful, I appreciate, but been there, done that, thank you.

For me the fear building in relation to this operation is the fear of anaesthetic. I don't understand it and I know it can be very dangerous. However, I know in my heart of hearts that I will go through with this operation, despite all my doubts and questions, because to me it will close this episode of breast cancer.

Monday 25 February

I registered today for a place in the London Marathon. If I can handle breast cancer I can certainly handle the matter of a small twenty-six mile run – I mean, how hard can this be?

Fingers crossed!

Tuesday 26 February

This time last year I was bald. And now it looks positively unkempt. Very pleased with my hairy look but think I should consider using the hairbrush more.

Friday 29 February

Well what an interesting day!

I am one of those people who sits, frustratingly, between a rock and a hard place when it comes to money.

The government cannot help me because I am freelance. The various cancer funds cannot help me because I have savings and therefore do not qualify for any grants. I only have the savings because I remortgaged my house to create the funds I would need to keep a roof over my head.

Frustratingly I am given telephone numbers of organisations who say they can help but cannot. I have given up jobs to fight for my life and yet I can get nothing back in return to help me. How can this be? Money does not grow on trees at the best of times, but least of all when you are unable to work because of an illness.

I had a long chat with BBC Radio Solent this morning. They are running a campaign entitled the 100 Lives project which follows the lives of one hundred ordinary local people over the period of one year. This ground-breaking project offers a unique insight into life in the twenty-first century, and they have chosen me to be a part of it.

Monday 3 March

I went on my first visit to BBC Radio Solent this morning. I was very nervous as I don't remember ever being on radio before. It is incredibly weird to be chatting to just one person in a room but to know that there are hundreds out there listening.

I spoke of my experience with breast cancer with candid honesty, and with help and encouragement from the team I was able to explain my experiences and my nerves for next week – when I am due to undergo my reconstructive surgery.

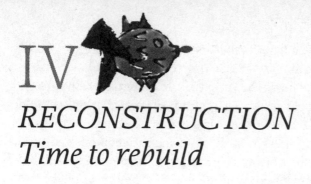

IV

RECONSTRUCTION
Time to rebuild

Wednesday 5 March 2008

... and the humiliating experiences just keep on coming!

I spent this afternoon at the Salisbury District Hospital attending a pre-op assessment in preparation for my reconstruction operation next Friday. I was confronted by a nurse wielding two large cotton buds the size of chopsticks. She was collating various bits of information required before entering hospital.

It was an emotional meeting. I cried, again, because I still don't like hospitals and I am still frightened of the anaesthetic, but the nurse was very good and calmed me down. She must hate people like me, but you would never have known. Anyway, just to complete the day, I was then sent off to be photographed naked from the waist up. I must admit I shall be delighted when I can walk into a room and leave my top on!

Friday 7 March

In less than one week I shall be issued with my new puppies! Noseless ones! I will undergo a right prophylactic mastectomy followed by bilateral reconstructive surgery with a latissimus dorsi flap, and today on the news I learned that women in my position are not being treated fairly and are not being offered reconstructive surgery at the time of mastectomy. A consultant onco-surgeon was shouting the odds about not being able to meet government targets. I was stunned! He of all people should realise that not every patient is suitable for reconstructive surgery at the time of the mastectomy. Each patient is different, and there are many reasons and complications that may prevent that operation taking place at the same time. The reason I have had to wait eighteen months since my first mastectomy is because I have had to undergo radiotherapy and, as a slim woman with small breasts my reconstruction will involve silicone implants – and it is not possible to undergo radiotherapy with silicone implants because (in layman's terms) they block the radiotherapy beams getting to the chest wall and thus reduce the chance of the radiotherapy being successful.

After completing my radiotherapy last year I had to wait at least six months before being able to undergo further surgery on the affected skin, which brought me to January 2008. I am one example of the many reasons that exist for not undergoing reconstructive surgery at the outset. Not least the fact that some women don't want it at that time but may discover, some years later, that they would quite like to feel complete again and apply for surgery in those later years.

Personally, I have thought long and hard about having this operation. I mean it isn't necessary – unlike the first mastectomy this operation is not life-saving.

I used to believe the old adage of 'if it isn't broken, then don't fix it!' So why am I putting my body through what, on the surface, appears to be quite unnecessary major surgery? The simple answer is that I *am* broken and I *do* need fixing. I am still a work-in-progress. Having lived with one breast for eighteen months I will be delighted to have two once again.

So after much soul searching I finish today content in the knowledge that I have made the correct decision.

Thursday 13 March

A very fidgety night was followed this morning by the unnerving feeling of almost passing out. My head was giddy and my arms felt like heavy weights. I felt drained and sick and unable to dress myself.

You see, today was check-in day at the hospital. We were required at the hospital in the mid-afternoon and I needed to pack, but I felt unprepared and was not willing to face up to today's challenge.

Rich did his thing – he pushed me onwards and ignored my behaviour. I think this was a good thing, although I could have done with a cuddle.

We arrived on time, a look of abject fear on my face that was read instantly by the ward administrator who was a lovely bubbly woman and who smiled a warm comforting smile and suggested that I should go down to pathology to get my blood test done as the ward, and all the individual pods within it, were undergoing their weekly deep clean. We wandered off and discovered the most amazing phlebotomists who, despite my collapsed and unresponsive veins due to my chemotherapy, managed to extract sufficient blood with little or no discomfort. We returned to Laverstock Ward and were sent to my pod.

With my head bowed, not wanting to look around me, I shuffled reluctantly into my pod of six and found my bed, tucked away in the corner. Together Rich and I sat talking of anything but where we were. We were advised to await the arrival of Mr Whitworth, my surgeon, and my anaesthetist. Fortunately, Mr Whitworth appeared promptly and saw the look of fear on my face. Together we discussed briefly what would be happening, and on his departure he suggested we go down to the local pub and have some supper and try to relax, but to return by nine.

My anaesthetist was with us within the hour and I proceeded to burst into tears the minute she walked in! Pathetic I know, but that is how I feel. I had to explain to the poor girl that it wasn't personal.

She was a sailor herself, so we talked about familiar things.

After dinner in the local pub – with a large glass of wine which I was permitted – we returned to the hospital. Rich tucked me in and I was left alone. The lights were out and the place was eerie. I could hear the nurses shuffling around quietly. I lay as still as possible on my bed, my mind racing, terrified as usual of what was to come. I looked down at my chest and though that this would be the last time I would see myself with one boob. Hurray! When this all began in October 2006 little did I know that it would be almost eighteen months before I would have two boobs once again.

Friday 14 March

I have completed three phases of this cancer treatment. Phase One: the Mastectomy... Phase Two: Chemotherapy... Phase Three: Radiotherapy. And finally, after eighteen months of approaching life the mono-boob way, I embarked on my final phase this morning – Phase Four: the Reconstruction.

As dawn broke the nurses put stockings on my lower legs to help my circulation, my pyjamas were changed for a stunning medical gown, and I was given a pre-med. Rich turned up and we were left alone for a while for me to calm down and relax.

Feeling very dozy, I remember being wheeled down the ward and along the corridor to the operating theatre with Rich clutching my hand. Lying on my back on the cart in the anteroom I studied the ceiling intently. People were talking to me yet I heard nothing. I was given some anaesthetic and slowly lost consciousness. I remember nothing else.

I awoke at around tea time, starving actually. I couldn't move and was hooked up to some drip or other. I turned my head and saw Rich sitting beside me, patiently reading a book and holding my left hand. I squeezed his hand gently and he looked over at me and smiled. I tried to talk, to tell him I love him, but I didn't have the energy.

As I dozed, Rich read. I watched him through my slumber as he sat beside me. Later in the evening Rich left me to sleep. I lay there alone once again and looked down at my chest which was covered in bandages. I thought about how I had today continued in my quest to donate to the NHS as much of my body as possible and had handed over my one remaining boob as a gift, undergoing the much-anticipated right prophylactic mastectomy followed by a bilateral reconstruction. A good deal from my perspective, I think, as they appear to have built me two new matching boobs which are a little larger and heavier than before (*well, why not!*). I just hope the new puppies fit into that lovely wedding dress that is being made for me in Singapore.

I do feel delighted to finally close the door on what I hope will be an end to this little journey. According to the medical team it began some eighteen months ago, but for me the nightmare began twenty months earlier, when I first tried to get the discharge from my left nipple taken seriously.

A prophylactic mastectomy reduces the likelihood of recurrence of breast cancer in my body by ninety-eight per cent, apparently. For me it was sensible to have taken such drastic action – removing the healthy right breast. If there is any way in which I can reduce the chances of repeating the past eighteen months then I will do it. When you have been butchered the way I have been, undergone chemotherapy and radiotherapy to control, dismiss and prevent the recurrence of such an unpleasant, deceitful disease, then why stop just before the final hurdle?

As I lay in my bed, my head dozy as I recovered from the anaesthetic, I dwelt on the statistics that eight out of ten women survive breast cancer with today's advances in modern medicine. The truth is that the rest of that quote is 'for five years'. Was I going through all this just to survive another five years? Should I not be running around enjoying myself without the forthcoming pain and discomfort of tomorrow whilst I have the chance? I will never know the answer to that, as I do not remember the rest of that thought.

Saturday 15 March

Why don't they listen? They say you know your own body better than anyone else does, so why don't they listen when you tell them something?

Blood tests. Five people, all doctors, and all think they can manage to take blood. All fail. Despite my telling them that my veins have toughened and are unresponsive as a result of my chemotherapy they seem surprised that they are unable to take blood from my right arm. Confirming that my veins have collapsed, I suggest that they try using smaller needles.

What a terrific way to be woken up. However, after the excitement of the doctors' visit I decided to go for a dawn wee on the commode this morning, which was highly embarrassing. I don't remember the last time I needed help to go to the loo, and in a room full of people too. It is true that cancer humbles you.

Anyway, after huge success on the commode I requested that I be left to sit in my chair to wait for the imminent arrival of my breakfast rather than returned to my bed. With rather concerned faces the nurses left me, as requested, bolt upright on my plastic chair tucked away in my corner. However, unsurprisingly, I was forced to call for help and returned, tail between my legs, to my bed. I was feeling incredibly light-headed and slightly sick and needed to lie down. This, I discover, was not surprising – as it turns out the operation took eight hours and I did not return to my pod until much later than I expected the previous evening. I had been out of surgery a little over twelve hours and whilst the nurses were delighted to see positive recovery they were highly doubtful that I would manage breakfast in that chair, but were wise enough not to argue with a very determined individual.

I was forced to eat humble pie until lunchtime, when I tried again to sit in the chair – this time with much success.

I had a breakthrough later today. As if by magic, as my watch beeped on the hour of noon, I worked out how to sit up in bed without using the mechanics of the bed as a lever and without the necessity to buzz the nurses' station for assistance. I used the circulation stockings that I was being forced to wear due to my immobility. I grabbed hold of these stockings at the thigh and pulled against them, and managed to pull myself up. I know I was buggering the DVT-reducing properties of the incredibly tight bed stockings but that didn't seem important to me at the time as I regained my independence. That was just brilliant!

I had many visitors today, which was wonderful. My little pod was very busy as Rich turned up with my friend Gail, and they were swiftly followed by my folks, immediately upsetting the two-visitors-only rule. Clearly I am very important!

Sunday 16 March

Last night was very frustrating as I found myself unable to get comfortable. As the operation had required two large incisions in both my left and right latissimus dorsi muscles – the two large back muscles that play a vital part in holding you upright – I was unable to lie back to sleep comfortably so found myself devising a plan to support myself with excessive amounts of pillows. This was a huge success but for a limited amount of time, and after a couple of hours I was woken by an intense nagging ache across the back which I was unable to calm. Drugs were not available until the early morning drug run so I remained awake.

In a desperate attempt to entertain myself whilst lying pinned to my bed I watched with interest the night shift pottering around the ward clutching *huge* torches, shining them into each bed, checking on their sleeping occupants. They looked like enormous fireflies.

Needless to say I was very ready for dawn. Fidgety and bored,

I leapt out of bed after receiving my first drugs of the day and having had my drains changed, to go for a walk. I wanted to stretch the old leggies – but I made sure I was back in time for my much needed and previously ordered breakfast of Marmite on toast, orange juice and apple.

The morning dragged as usual, and with the assistance of Columbo on my hospital television I raced towards more food at noon and on towards visiting time. My lovely Rich arrived and we made a break for it. I was helped out of bed, out of the pod and off down the corridor, past the new as yet unpacked dishwasher that had been there since we arrived stacked by the kitchen area of the ward, and out of the ward. This was my first foray into the unknown and as yet unexplored corridors of Floor 4 of the Salisbury District Hospital, and on the arm of my fiancé, with drains in tow of course, we hopped into the lift.

After a brief escape we returned to my six-bed pod and shortly after were joined by a dear friend, Carol. She is a local lass who popped in armed with one grape, one plum and a small stuffed cow. I understand that the cow was the animal of choice because they have udders and I had just been issued with a completely new set of udders too – apparently! How lovely.

The endless rounds of tea continued as our friends John and Karen, Rach and my sister Kate swelled the numbers in my pod, and we were banished to the day room.

Monday 17 March

I am beginning to feel like a caged animal, spending much of the morning fidgeting, sitting around waiting for the hordes to be let in to visit early afternoon. Being in hospital is a little like being in a zoo.

However, another success in the independence stakes as I managed to wash my own hair this morning. The last time my rapidly lengthening blonde locks saw shampoo and water was last Thursday, before the operation, so sporting a rather creased set of pink floral pyjamas, four rapidly expanding drain sacks stuffed into a rather grotty hospital pillow case, *to spare my blushes* (!), a pair of pink spotty slippers that were just a tiny bit too small, as my mother had put them through the wash and they had shrunk, I pottered off to the bathroom containing the walk-in shower facility and spent an eternity trying to work out the best way to hold the shower hose, hold my drain pillow case, hold my sponge and then actually wash myself without getting myself wet from the waist up! Challenging indeed, but the sense of achievement when I burst out through the door some thirty minutes later was enormous. Further proof that my stubbornness has been vital throughout this whole cancer experience.

Tuesday 18 March

And so begin the endless rounds of tea once more. Six am brings a shift change, drug round and tea trolley. What a busy morning we have when most of the country are still asleep. By breakfast we are all exhausted again. We patients have been poked, checked, tested and emptied.

Why do hospitals insist on such an early wake-up call? By the time we are allowed any visitors in the early afternoon we have all done a full eight-hour day. I glance around my pod and wonder about my companions. We are a fun but varied collection, and we are without doubt the noisiest pod. The woman next door to me keeps herself to herself, sits quietly reading her newspaper, day in, day out without a visitor in sight, but there are two ladies in here with me who have been with me the whole time. The lovely lady opposite me has also undergone reconstructive surgery, and in the bed next to her is a wonderful old lady with such a great character. We three chat regularly.

Wednesday 19 March

A momentous occasion took place today. My wounds were healing sufficiently for me to be allowed to have the back two drains removed. Hurray! The contents of the little pink cloth bag I carry around have reduced, as has the weight. Carrying around four drain bags with fluid in is quite heavy work.

I am told that I can go home when I have had the final two removed. The drains are removing fluid from my wound sites. It was a large operation requiring them to cut into my muscles, causing bleeding, and I am to remain in hospital until this bleeding has stopped. As long as the drains remain in me, I remain in here!

Thursday 20 March

The more I gain confidence in my recent operation the more I am prepared to read about what exactly they did to me. My mind runs riot with visions of being pulled and pushed around on the operating table, turned over, sat up, laid back down again and generally being treated like a punch bag.

I remember the first meeting with Mr Whitworth and remember coming home and researching further into the details of silicone implants on the internet to learn about the foreign body that I was to have sewn into me, but it was decided that I should not read too much beforehand. That was probably a wise move knowing me. However, now, as time moves on past the operation date itself I feel strong enough to learn more.

Together with details of what they actually did to me in the operating theatre I have learnt about silicone implants. I have learnt that they can occasionally leak fluid. The chances of the breast implant leaking increases over time. Most implants that have been in place for between ten and fifteen years have some leakage, but it's usually insignificant. The breast will reduce in size if the implant is leaking but this leak is harmless. Apart from the size change of the breast, these leaks can show up on an ordinary MRI scan, or sometimes on a regular x-ray.

Today is ward deep-cleaning day. Whilst the ward is cleaned daily, once a week a full deep clean takes place. One side of the pod is moved over to the other side. Each bed, side table and chair – and patient installed in the bed too if necessary – is wheeled over to the other side of the pod and the place is thoroughly disinfected from top to bottom.

Saturday 22 March

Home James, and don't spare the horses!

Finally! I have been discharged – although I have cheated. I still have the two remaining drains in place but I am going nuts pacing the wards and probably driving the nurses spare. It has been an incredibly frustrating and fidgety ten days, I was feeling ever more like a caged animal and I desperately wanted to take the new puppies home. I think the nurses were also glad to see me leave today, actually. As many of you will appreciate, keeping me still is a huge challenge for anyone. It is great to be home.

So, boobs! Two of them again. It is a little extreme, having them removed, just to avoid the unpleasant and uncomfortable feeling of a mammogram – but for me my peace of mind is priceless.

I was just settling into the sofa again, and half expecting to embark on another prolonged period enthroned there. But Rich knew better, and after dropping off my bag we headed out to take the puppies for a walk. A gentle stroll towards the village but not managing to get to there. Each day I aim to get further.

Monday 24 March

Having pretty much stubbed out the opportunity for breast cancer to recur in my body directly, by removing both breasts, I now focus on the potential recurrence of a cancer as a result of my original breast cancer – secondary breast cancer.

The vulnerable areas of the body that are susceptible to breast cancer recurrence are the lung, the liver, the brain and the bones. All of these have a high risk of attack as a result of a primary development of breast cancer.

I am running the fine line between neurosis and lackadaisical. Was that headache this morning the beginning of brain cancer as a result of a previous diagnosis of breast cancer or simply a regular headache? My tiredness this afternoon – was that a symptom of bone metastases or a result of staying up late watching a movie? My backache surely cannot be the first sign of bone metastases, surely it is because I am holding myself in such a peculiar stiff fashion as a result of the drains that are still stitched into my body?

Questions like this roam around in my head, and I am beginning to become paranoid.

Before being diagnosed with breast cancer I would have thought nothing of being a little dozy one Sunday afternoon after a late Saturday night – but now I imagine it to be the beginning of something quite different!

Tuesday 25 March

Finally! The flow of fluids from my wound sites has reduced sufficiently for me to return to hospital with Rich today to have my remaining front drains removed. It was a truly uncomfortable and weird feeling as the nurse pulled out two feet or more of clear pipe that had been stuffed into my body and stitched into place. It doesn't hurt but it can feel very odd, as you can imagine. There is the risk of them getting caught, heaven knows on what, as they are pulled out, but fortunately mine were behaving.

Wednesday 26 March

With the removal of my drains yesterday I was able to embark on a full head-to-toe shower. Finally I could stand under the shower head and not worry about getting anything wet that I shouldn't – and it felt fabulous. I stood there for ages.

I got out of the shower and looked at myself in my full glory. I am a rather sorry sight but I am alive. I didn't dwell too long on the sight in the mirror.

My new little puppies don't have noses. No nipples. I look a little like a mannequin, I think.

I decided to do some more homework this afternoon into *exactly* what they had been doing with me and my body over the past ten days.

In medicine, a *pedicle* refers to the part of a tissue graft that remains attached to the donor site, and so because the latissimus dorsi flap is not completely disconnected from its source at any point in the reconstruction surgery it is classified as a 'pedicle flap'. During latissimus dorsi flap breast reconstruction, a tunnel is created beneath the skin from the back muscle to the breast area. The surgeon transfers the flap – an oval section of skin, some fat and part of the latissimus dorsi muscle – and slides it around through this tunnel under the skin under the arm to the breast area. Blood vessels remain attached whenever possible but if any have been cut during the procedure then these are reconnected with microsurgery to blood vessels in the chest area. The tissue is then shaped into a natural-looking breast and sewn into place and an implant is also inserted during the same operation to form the breast content.

There are of course pros and cons to this operation and I note these – but it is a little like shutting the stable door after the horse has bolted.

- Plus – Many breast surgeons like this procedure because the flap is easily slipped around to the front, through a short tunnel in the skin, and put into position. Generally this procedure produces excellent results with few complications.

- Minus – The skin on your back has a slightly darker colour and texture to that of breast skin, but the difference is almost unnoticeable. (*I would agree with that.*)

- Minus – Latissimus dorsi also results in some back asymmetry (unevenness in the appearance of your back). Usually, though, back function and strength aren't affected.

When I look at myself now and think how I looked before I consider these to be small concerns. Everything in perspective. Alive, two boobs and an element of my femininity returned.

Thursday 27 March

I received a lovely note today from an Australian friend who had been on my Sydney to Hobart crew. A nurse herself, she was congratulating me on reaching the final stage of what I have regularly referred to as my cancer nightmare. I have been thinking about her words. She wondered how anyone could possibly imagine or understand what I have been through. Apparently I am an inspiration, which is lovely to hear – but I am not really an inspiration, I am just desperate to stay alive. I would do anything to stay alive.

She says that God only deals out to us what we can handle – apparently. An interesting thought. Have I handled it? I am not sure. I do know that I am seventeen months further on than I ever imagined I would be.

I took my puppies out for another walk today. It was a bit drizzly actually and I wondered whether I should have got a towel ready so that they could be rubbed down on my return.

I am told that early training will be crucial to keep them under control, otherwise they could develop minds of their own, sneaking out when they shouldn't. Perhaps training them to catch sticks will prove to be the most challenging!

Friday 28 March

My new puppies have created quite a stir and I have received quite an array of advice on how to handle them. I have had to explain on numerous occasions, however, that these puppies are *not* for stroking!

Monday 31 March

I had an interview with the *Southern Echo* today. They are doing an article on me, which is great. The reporter was lovely.

A friend asked me why I was prepared to talk to strangers about something so personal. Well, two reasons really. Firstly because when I was looking for answers at the beginning, or perhaps looking for someone I could talk to or listen to about their experiences, there was no-one apart from the medical team – who spoke from a medical viewpoint, emotionless, about a hugely personal and terrifying ordeal – and secondly, I think it is also a way for me to come to terms with what has happened

Tuesday 1 April

I am not loving the new puppies today! They are heavier and my back muscles are still weak from the operation. I have ached more today than I have throughout this whole cancer nightmare. There will be some who say it is because I have moved around too much and not spent enough time sitting still as instructed by the medical team, but there will be others who will remember that I have undergone major surgery, a mere two weeks ago, and that this is absolutely normal. Time is the healer and patience is an absolute must. Clearly I had lost my box of patience somewhere and have been delving too quickly into my box of 'I must do everything myself – now!'

Just looking at my chest hurts today. The internal bruising where my drains were, the tops of my new boobs, the incision marks at the donor site – all of me feels just a little bit sorry for myself today. What have I done?

Today is the sixtieth anniversary of the NHS and we learn that the cost of a prescription is rising and is dependent on your postcode. The NHS motto is 'Healthcare free at the point of use' – oh really.

I have been prescribed a life-saving drug that I must take daily for five years and I have to pay for it. It is not a luxury, neither is it a choice, it is life-saving and along with many other patients in my position we do not have the choice – but neither do we have the help.

Thursday 10 April

I had my first interview with BBC Radio Solent since my operation. I enjoy my chats with Charlie on air, and with her production team, and I hope that people who have been diagnosed with breast cancer can gain some inspiration and encouragement from me. Alternatively my story might help those who know someone with breast cancer to understand and communicate with her, and help them to handle their friend/family member, because it can sometimes be hard for them to know where to start.

I don't think I have anything particular to add to the details that I have already given to the listeners about my cancer except that this reconstruction has made me feel whole again – physically, I am a complete woman again. It feels like I have completed my circle. I believe that if I hadn't had the surgery I would always feel like I had not finished with cancer, if you know what I mean. However, it is not all that simple – despite my making the decision in November 2006 to have this right prophylactic mastectomy and full bilateral reconstruction at the end of all the treatment, I have spent much time over the past year worrying about whether I should go ahead with the reconstruction operation, because essentially it was not a necessity, and I wondered whether I should put myself at risk or put myself through something so major. The truth is that I knew I was always going to go through with the reconstruction, but as usual this disease plays with your mind and there is always that moment of panic just before something major when you think perhaps you shouldn't do it to yourself. I was fit and healthy and sailing again in anger and living life to the full. So why bother?

However, the operation is over and was a huge success – but I do still look at myself and wonder what I have done, because it can take some getting used to.

Friday 25 April

I rather foolishly took my new puppies for their first sail today, six weeks after the reconstruction operation. Feeling great, I hoisted the mainsail and my back complained. I went below to nurse my wounds feeling very silly. When they say six months to recover they mean six months and not six weeks! However, I am not very good at sitting still and wanted to go back to work as soon as possible – but my job is not the average job, I guess. Back to the gentle walks and no lifting. How on earth I thought I would ever be able to run the marathon this weekend, so soon after this operation, I do not know.

Friday 9 May

I went into BBC Radio Solent again today to discuss my reconstruction. I described my feelings of closure of my battle with the blowfish and how amazing it feels, even at this early stage, to have two boobs and a return, despite the healing process still to come, of my femininity.

I know I grinned from ear to ear.

Sunday 22 June

I put my new puppies through their first challenging physical test yesterday. Rich and I held our stag and hen celebration this weekend. Our 'stench' – stag, hen and munch – was a joint affair consisting of an energetic and very muddy army assault course, then a raft-building competition, followed by a lively murder mystery dinner. It was wonderful to spend the weekend with so many friends, and with Rupert and Leanne, but I don't think my breast surgeon will be best pleased with me when I next see him!

Thursday 10 July

Our wedding is only two days away.

I went on a final visit to BBC Radio Solent. With my wedding a part of my story for their 100 Lives project I was delighted to go and see them, but this time I took both my ten-year-old soon-to-be stepdaughter Hannah and the ever-faithful Gilly. It was great fun. Han spoke for most of the interview but Gilly was rendered somewhat silent. I am not sure if she was terrified or just being polite, but it was very amusing to note such silence from such a chatty young lady!

I was given a super send-off from the studio and a lovely pressie from the team, who have become such familiar faces.

We returned to Chateau Pontin-Falk. Best man, umpteen members of the Australian contingent and two further bridesmaids had packed bags and cars with everything but the kitchen sink and so a household of people bundled themselves into five cars and the road trip to my parents began, with one car peeling off to collect the cake.

A little under an hour later we arrived in Sutton, the small, beautiful South Downs village that is to play host to the circus. Rich's family have moved into a fabulously converted old tractor shed which now boasts all mod cons, which we nicknamed Australia House, and the wedding party of bridesmaids and groomsmen was, perhaps unwisely, moved into the local pub. Family Pontin laid claim to my folks' house, and the marquee had taken over the lawn.

It was brilliant!

The rehearsal at the church had been arranged for teatime and it was quite frankly a disaster with people giggling and messing around. After a stern reprimand from David, our lovely vicar, we completed the preparations for Saturday and returned to the bedlam at the house.

A relaxed and chilled dinner for twenty-five was held around one long table placed on the dance floor of the marquee and we celebrated into the early hours, with the little people heading to bed not long before the adults.

Friday 11 July

It was a slow and sluggish start for many of the party after a late night. My mother had trundled down to the church with Jack and Georgia, my niece and nephew, who had been up early and were followed by Ann, a truly talented lady who was to do the flowers. She led a team from the village and they worked tirelessly to decorate this fabulous church. It looked amazing.

The Australian contingent took all the small children off to a castle and a picnic for the day, and final preparations continued.

Daddy and one of Rich's sisters decided to cut the hedges and stay out of the way too. An excellent move, I think.

With everything as under control as it can be the day before hosting a wedding of one hundred and twenty guests, my parents moved the circus down to the village pub, which we took over, and our families were joined by many friends from the village who know us all very well. After all, this is a village that has taken on the terrifying breast cancer nightmare with my parents, offering support and love when they needed it – and this wonderful celebration brings relief and thanks too.

An early-ish night for all. I wandered home holding Rupert's arm and clutching the diamond bracelet that Rich had given me this evening to wear tomorrow. 'Chosen to help you sparkle, Em.'

Saturday 12 July

Wedding Day.

I snuck out of the house for a run with Gilly, who had rather foolishly offered to come with me – though she hadn't bargained with first being videoed by my over-excitable brother, who followed me around with his camera from the moment I woke up with the twins going nuts running around us. My excitement was uncontrollable at this stage.

I am back in the running shoes after a break on strict instructions from my reconstruction surgeon to give the puppies a chance to settle in, and I have always been determined not to let our wedding day stop this enthusiasm. Gilly and I talked between trying to breathe as we ran through the village and out past the church. I admitted that I never thought today would arrive.

We returned to find the kitchen awash with flowers as Ann and Mummy began the six bouquets and numerous buttonholes for the bridal party. Upstairs, a bedroom had been designated the hair salon, and the girls one by one were washed, brushed and styled. I was to go last and paced the floors.

My father was last seen in the garden – sweeping!

As the house fell silent Daddy and I finally left the building suitably, and politely, late and were driven by my brother in a beautiful shiny black car. Unlike my brother and father, I am not a petrolhead and therefore couldn't tell you what the car *was* but I know what it *wasn't*. My father owns a beautiful bright red V8 Morgan and I was determined to arrive at my wedding in this stunning sports car. However, it was pointed out to me on numerous occasions in the build-up to the wedding day that I wouldn't get into it in a dress. Mother has enough trouble when wearing trousers let alone attempting it in a cream, very straight and very long wedding dress and full-length veil. This advice I refused to heed, but I was quietly and effectively overruled when Rupert turned up in the black number.

I was beaten. And they were right. But don't tell anyone! I could hear the bells ringing as we drove the small distance through the village and were met by David, the vicar, and my bridesmaids. As we walked up the church path and positioned ourselves at the door I could see Loz through the entrance smiling at me. I wanted to cry and was shaking like a leaf. My father held my hand so tightly and I squeezed his in response.

With the smiles on the faces of my friends and family beaming at me I was led down the aisle grinning from ear to ear. I wanted desperately to remember everything. After finding my mother with my eyes I moved my gaze to the front and to the man I was to marry. Rich's eyes beamed and his warm smile was just perfect.

After a beautiful ceremony with a fabulously funny reading written and performed by another of Rich's sisters, with reference to marriage as a pair of slippers made from elastic bands, Rich and I left the church to the immortal words of Stevie Wonder's 'Signed, sealed, delivered I'm yours' and the entire party strolled back through the village in the sunshine behind a Scottish piper. It was magnificent.

Tears of laughter and emotion took over as my father and now new husband both spoke. They touched briefly on the battle with the blowfish, an issue that was not to be dwelt on today of all days but must be mentioned – after all, it has, to date, formed such a huge part of our lives together.

Rich and I led the onslaught on the dance floor, to Robbie Williams' beautiful rendition of 'Mack the Knife'. Wrapped in my husband's arms it was as if no-one else was in the room.

Exhausted and happy, Rich and I left the party at midnight and were shepherded off to a stunning converted vintage Victorian railway carriage located in the forest where we spent our first night, with champagne and each other, as Mr and Mrs Richard Falk. I don't ever remember feeling this happy.

Sunday 13 July

We returned this morning to mayhem once more, as today my parents were hosting the families and the village. Drinks and canapés on the lawn preceded our rather unusual and spectacular James-Bond-style lunchtime exit. Mark was a good friend of mine from my legal days in London, a senior banking lawyer by profession – but he is a helicopter pilot, and he gave us the most amazing wedding present. We were to leave by helicopter.

We were whisked away to stay in a friend's house in the south of France for a couple of days' rest and alone time, with a proper honeymoon to follow one day when we can afford one – cancer is an expensive illness.

Thursday 17 July

Our first steps across the threshold into our home were met by a house full of people. Most of Rich's family were still there with his children. It was a lovely reception and we wined and dined with Ranna, Johnny, Trish, the children and Addie regaling us with stories of the wedding itself and the past few days. It is always interesting to hear about a party, or in this case wedding, that you are hosting from someone else's perspective! Many things took place at our wedding that I was unaware of, I discovered this evening.

With the sad departure to the airport of the last Australian at the end of this week, Rich, myself and the children are scheduled to disappear to Dorset for a few days' camping before the children have to return to the USA. I just hope the English weather behaves – but I shall be packing my thermals.

Saturday 5 September

I have developed a ridiculous and terrible, uncontrollable fear of flying, so today I attended an official Fear of Flying course organised by British Airways. This course is offered by many of the airlines to their customers and gives some information about the principles of flying together with an explanation of the basic psychology behind the human reaction of fear.

Apparently it is lack of control that I fear, and it is something that is quite normal after a traumatic experience such as an encounter with a life-threatening situation. After I broke myself I was forced to give myself to a team of specialists who would fix me (like a Lego figure broken by a child), and when the doctors returned my body with my life fixed I then became very reluctant to let anyone risk breaking it.

When I am sailing I am the skipper of a yacht. I am in control, I am responsible for my own life and for those of others. When I am driving a car I am at the wheel and in control, and therefore responsible for my life and those of others, but when I am flying I am handing my life to another person, the pilot, in effect putting it at risk without playing a part – and that scares me.

Of course, I understand the principles of flying as they are the same as sailing – based on lift – but I found the psychology very interesting and will wait to see if I can get a grip next time I take a flight.

Friday 26 September

As a breast cancer patient with no natural breasts any more, I am told that breast cancer, should it metastasise, will do so in the form of secondary cancer in the lung, liver, brain or bone. These are very difficult organs to monitor, I decided, as I cannot see them, not like you can see a breast. They are also inside the body, and if any returning blowfish were missed then it would be very difficult for the medical team to deal with. With that in mind I went in to cancerphobic overdrive and organised a full-body bone scan, and today I shot off to have my scan dragging the ever-faithful Jen along with me to another medical appointment. Poor girl – she seems to get the rough ones, as she was the one who had to deal with me during my head-shaving episode. This time she was dragged along to another medical appointment by her neurotic and pathetic friend, who proceeds to cry her way through each visit!

After being injected with a small dose of radiation dye type stuff I was plonked in front of what looked like a small television set and, with both Jen and the camera operator in the room with me, my whole body was photographed. I was moved from position to position with the camera clicking away, reacting to the injection fluid and seeking any problems that might be lurking inside my bones.

Today's scan may not have been necessary but it did me no harm and settled my mind. I remain on full alert – and ever so slightly neurotic about cancer returning.

Monday 17 November

I flew out to join my yacht today for the start of another transatlantic race. The ARC is fast becoming very significant to me, as it was the race I missed two years ago and the one I skippered last year, one year after the diagnosis. Once again I would make it to the start line. My emotions for this race will never change. My attendance on this start line is a benchmark for my survival.

Big Spirit is the name of my boat this year. A bright orange seventy-two-foot round-the-world racing yacht – and I love her. A yacht I know very well as I learned to sail on her in 2003 when, as a non-sailor, I undertook my first transatlantic yacht race. I went on to spend the following three years working on the large fleet that belonged to the Challenge Business, a sailing organisation conceived and run by Sir Chay Blyth.

She is a fifty-tonne steel yacht designed to take the worst the oceans can offer – the rigours of upwind ocean racing – and I feel very comfortable on board. However, this is a yacht with a difference. Now privately owned, she has been updated slightly and been given air conditioning, flat-screen televisions and a washing machine – I have never crossed an ocean in such luxury. She is barely recognisable from the workhorse that housed an eighteen-man crew.

This race is what we call in the industry a downwind race, with the winds coming from behind most of the way – so for this heavy monster it is going to be a challenge, but a delightful one.

Sunday 23 November

After a week of extensive preparation and sail training we slipped lines at 1030 hours this morning and motored out of the marina to head for the 'playground' – an area just off the east coast of Gran Canaria – to hoist sails and get into the swing of things. Due to our size and weight and the crowded start line we opted for a simple sail plan. We hoisted a full main with only one foresail – the yankee number 1. The second forward sail, the staysail, was left in the sail locker to make life easier on the start line. (*For those of you who don't speak yacht, the yankee is the sail at the very front of the boat, more commonly known as a jib between friends, and the staysail is the sail just back from the yankee.*)

We tacked and gybed around the start area, assessing the line and marking out our intended start and checking the angles and the time it took to reach the line so that our approach could be effective and fast. After putting in a few tacks and gybes, with the cheers and foghorns of spectator boats ringing in our ears, the horn for the ten-minute countdown sounded and the adrenaline began to pump. I looked around the boat and the smiles on the faces of my crew became broader and broader. Their wait to begin their first transatlantic race was almost over. All eyes were outside the boat checking for competitors making a beeline for the bright orange boat. Bang – the five-minute gun and we were in the thick of it. Fortunately people were clearing a path for us as we powered along the edge of the start line, which made our life easier, and as the final countdown to the race start blasted out over the VHF radio we were all in position: 8, 7, 6, 5, 4, 3, 2, 1 – GO! Next stop St Lucia. The wait was over and the race was on!

Now then – I would like to introduce you to my crew – a fun and rowdy bunch – eleven of us in total. We cover three nationalities and a full spectrum of experience and character. Sadly our twelfth man had to leave us unexpectedly the day before race start and we remain a little lost without him. We hope to make him proud.

As we settled into our day, the race start over, the adrenaline of the start line easing a little, the troops began to relax and enjoy the sun and the beautiful breeze that was being kind to this heavy orange beast, propelling us at a very healthy eleven knots in the direction of Africa. All was well with the world.

I too settled into life on board and marvelled at my surroundings. Ambling from the double cabin I headed to the laundry room, being careful not to knock the tumble drier and washing machine as I went in, to rummage through one of the two freezers on board containing huge quantities of fresh, now frozen, meat and treats to retrieve a frozen Mars Bar. On my way back past the galley I stopped to collect some fresh fruit for a crew member and check the time on the microwave. I was just heading up on deck after taking time to select what to wear from an array of clothes I had been allowed to take with me on this trip and that is stored safely in a collection of boxes. I remember thinking how wonderful my permitted showers will be!

Now all this may seem completely normal for many of the ARC participants, but for me, on my umpteenth crossing of this ocean, this is the most luxurious. You must remember that the last time I sailed on board one of these yachts, of which there are twelve in the fleet, I was entering a round-the-world yacht race which was bound for the Southern Ocean where freeze-dried food and daily handfuls of vitamins and minerals to keep the body happy were the order of the day. Where cleanliness came in the form of four baby wipes per day and the choice of clothing was a dirty team T-shirt or the second, spare, hopefully slightly cleaner team T-shirt left in our one storage box. Microwaves, washing machines, fresh food, unlimited clothing – all very unusual items for me at sea. A very different experience, and what a treat! This is truly a luxuriously converted boat. I could get very used to it.

As we settled into the night watches the boat went quiet and on deck darkness fell. However, I was rudely awoken by the sharp movement of the boat and the calls from the on-deck watch to turn away from the wind. The boat kept turning, creating an unusual motion down below. Next I heard an exclamation and the boat tried to gybe – thank heavens for preventers! We were being targeted – a large fishing boat was making a beeline for us. We were fully lit and the boat had been spotted but to the on-deck watch's horror it turned at the last minute and went for us. With hearts pumping, our orange beast was manoeuvred into a safe position and calm ensued on deck – each crew member imagining what would have happened if ... A call placed on the VHF to all ARC boats in our vicinity ensured that all were aware of this crazy boat – which, as we turned, proceeded to play the same stunt on the yacht to our stern. Playing chicken with the two-hundred-and-forty-strong transatlantic racing and cruising fleets was clearly his game.

Tuesday 25 November

A beautiful crimson dawn broke this morning, and relief followed as the wind built. We had experienced an incredibly frustrating night with winds of just one knot at their least and a boat speed of 0.0 knots – and bearing in mind we weigh fifty tonnes that is not helpful in a yacht race. High hopes over breakfast with the wind blowing a fabulous twelve knots.

So today was kite day! An enormous spinnaker – the unmistakable bright orange of our boat and the size of a tennis court – was launched just after breakfast. The knitting that takes place around our decks to achieve this is quite spectacular, with each line having been carefully run so as to avoid carnage. Up went one of our enormous spinnaker poles, swiftly followed by the orange beast, and with the final drop of the yankee and pull of the sheet (*rope*) we were under kite and doing beautifully. The boat speed rose and with it the spirits of the crew as the arrival time in St Lucia went up to 9 December – as opposed to the rather soul-destroying mid-January which was predicted by our GPS during our night-time crawl.

Mother Watch today produced an array of wonderful foods including freshly baked scones with strawberry jam for afternoon tea. We were just missing the Cornish clotted cream! As part of Mother Watch you have a treat after all the cleaning and cooking, and that is a power shower. Hurray! Mother Watch I thought would be fun, but when I checked the rota that had been prepared I noted that my name did not appear and discovered that I was not scheduled to do Mother Watch – which means that I am not going to get a shower!

Panic over. It appears that a third person chosen by lucky dip will get to shower each day, and today was my day. So after high tea I pottered off to my hot shower, which was wonderful.

We are developing a boat language which, rather unnervingly, the crew all seem to have created and mastered, and it is only day three. The newest addition to our dictionary is 'twangled' – an American word used to describe the action of getting completely tangled up in a safety harness line with the only hope of extraction being to pirouette whilst lifting one leg. This I think would look more amusing if it were done to music!

On deck the crew learn how to fly, trim and eventually drop the kite, and after full instructions throughout the day the kite does us proud and makes some fantastic mileage for us. After another cracking offering from the galley we prepare to drop the kite, and with everyone in position – including a man dangling out over the ocean at the end of the aforementioned spinnaker pole – the call comes to 'spike and drop'. Down comes the kite in one fluid movement with no hitches, to be stuffed rather unceremoniously down below. The deck is re-rigged and down below the packing team begins the herculean task of sorting and packing the kite. This involves tying little pieces of black wool at regular two-foot intervals along the kite, which by this time has been manoeuvred into the shape of a sausage with two little legs running the length of the boat. All this preparation work must be done without creating a single twist, and all in a two-foot wide corridor. This is an art form which takes practice, and which the crew, by the end of the race, should have down to ten minutes – as opposed to the current time frame of just over an hour.

So night watches begin again and some people head off to their bunks. My team begin their duty at 2300 hours and we chat our way through four hours putting the world to rights, even resorting to naming our favourite television programmes – and all the time trying to achieve a boat speed that will make the rest of the crew proud of us. But by 3 am yawns are spotted and we are all desperate to go to bed.

So as we hand over to the 0300–0700 night watch we head off to bed, leaving the dawn patrol to find boat speed out of seven knots of breeze.

Wednesday 26 November

Dawn broke to produce another beautiful sunny day with crystal blue skies and the call for a kite launch. The big orange beastie went up again and stayed there – all day. The boat, driven and trimmed by the crew, propelled us in the direction of the Cape Verdes, humming along at perfectly respectable speeds of eight knots.

Once again we continued to eat – I swear this is the only transatlantic crossing where I will put on weight! After a hearty breakfast, tea and biscuits arrived mid-morning, then lunch – today wonderful bacon butties – followed by our standard afternoon tea and cake which arrived at 3 pm. Supper swiftly followed at 1740 hours. I couldn't move! We will all look like beached whales by the time we arrive in St Lucia. I think restraint is required.

This is proving to be a gentle race compared to the stormy episode of last year, with sunbathing the order of the day. However, we did have an energetic afternoon moving the spinnaker pole forward at least three inches – once. The troops seemed to separate into one-sex teams with the boys up first – one helm, one trimmer and one grinder – setting the girls a boat-speed target to chase. After hours of trading the play area between teams a cracking ten and a half knots was obtained and held by the boys before the kite was dropped just after supper, and I am pleased to report that the time it took to pack the kite was rapidly reduced this time to a healthy forty-five minutes – a race record!

Conversation continued throughout the day and was frankly rather risqué so I shall leave it on the boat where it belongs. Sadly not a boat in sight all day and no wildlife to play with either except for reports of little phosphorescing torpedoes playing on the bow at dusk. (*That's dolphins, for those who haven't had the pleasure of sailing at night.*) Once again the night watches settled into place, and for me a change of timing and a change of watch members. I took the 0300–0700 watch and once again conversation resorted to important issues – this time to include our top ten favourite movies, with *The Wizard of Oz* being named as a favourite. In amongst all the movie chitchat conducted by four people who eventually admitted to not really being movie watchers a top speed of twelve knots was reached. Content in our achievement, my watch handed over the helm and headed for their bunks.

Thursday 27 November

Last night saw the first hairy night of the race so far for the crew, with wind speeds topping twenty-three knots and a heavy sea state producing a roll that required an enormous amount of concentration when driving. We did, however, pull out a consistent boat speed of ten knots, which rapidly reduced our arrival time in the Caribbean. The once suspected prospect of spending Christmas and New Year on the boat bobbing around this pond has been shattered. Quite annoying, really, as a decision had just been made as to which crew member would become the best Christmas lunch in the absence of turkey.

Today was a very special day for two members of our crew in particular. It was Thanksgiving Day and the various (and numerous) offerings that appeared from the galley were American in flavour. Our American contingent took control of the galley and produced an array of American-accented meals and treats, and at high tea I was presented with a plate of cheese and salami – but as one half of the responsible adults on board I sadly had to forego the glass of wine that everyone else enjoyed. Before our Thanksgiving tea we made the crew work and asked them to put in a gybe to put us on a direct course for St. Lucia – with some terrific winds propelling us towards the rum.

As night-time drew close the wind built, and the decision to put a reef in the mainsail came in order to reduce the roll and make driving much easier in the dark. This was the first in-motion reef that the crew had undertaken, and it was executed with precision and speed. I was very impressed.

And so to bed for the other two watches, the Graveyard Shift and the Dawn Chorus, whilst the other watch kicked in – and kicked in it did!

The seas built and produced the most challenging helming to date. The night was pitch black with no horizon and no moon. Teamwork took hold, and with one crew member driving, one calling the apparent wind direction and one calling something else (which I couldn't quite make out from the comfort of my bunk!) they drove us admirably through a very unpleasant few hours. Thankfully the winds abated and by dawn the reef was shaken out and we resumed a very pleasant trade-wind course towards the finish line. Another day tomorrow and another wind pattern.

Friday 28 November

As the dust settled from last night I surveyed the scene of devastation on the deck. Coffee stains everywhere gave away the carnage of the early-evening watch struggling with the helm. Huge quartering seas and strong winds put them all to the test. An exhausted crew snuggled in their bunks now with my watch doing battle with an odd combination of lights. They sat off our port beam and appeared to show the lights of a trawler. We watched her on the radar move forward at twenty-one knots then back on a reciprocal course at six knots and yet she remained on our port beam. Eventually, as our courses were clearly converging, a VHF call was placed and a sorry sounding voice responded that they were in fact a sailing vessel in the ARC and had, during the rather hairy night, managed to jam their main half up, half down and had decided to wait for the seas to calm and dawn to arrive before attempting a fix. They told us that they were under motor. It was agreed that they would continue on course but would throttle back to ensure that we could pass unhindered, as we were still racing. At that, we wished them well and decided to shake out a reef. It had made life easier for us during the night but was now hindering our progress.

Sadly for the stricken yacht this involved us turning directly towards them, thus presenting a complete change of light sequence and resulting in a second, more panicked VHF communication with stricken yacht. They requested, with a little strain in the voice, our intentions – in reply to which I explained our movements and that we would resume our course in a couple of minutes.

All settled down and my watch enjoyed the dawn, fresh tea and a calmer sea state. Talk of kite hoisting rang out. As the sun peeped through a cotton-wool-cloud sky various items of clothing began to be removed. Two new 'mothers' stepped into the galley for the day to tend to our every catering need. A hand of bananas which had been forgotten and buried in the fruit and vegetable locker was beginning to make its presence known, and a suggestion of banana pancakes was proposed and approved.

The afternoon was fast and furious in the right direction and a relaxed crew soaked in the sun, read and generally chilled out. With dusk came the best meal on board yet – the mothers had excelled and produced a brilliant meal, raising the standards for the mothers in the days that are to follow.

It was, as usual, showers for the mothers. I managed to squeeze myself into the shower schedule somehow, which was lovely, and so I pottered off to my bunk. (Well, someone else's bunk actually – long story but suffice it to say that my nickname is 'Hobo' as I don't have a permanent bunk and sleep where and when I can – sobs of sympathy, please!)

Saturday 29 November

I must introduce you to my new friend. Since my arrival on board I have discovered a new toy at the chart table that was not here when I first sailed these boats in 2003. It is called the AIS navigation system and it is magic! It reveals all sorts of detail about the boat which is transmitting and I am slowly driving the crew up the wall with my new-found knowledge of any commercial boats larger than us in the vicinity. I can recite any number of bits of information to include their length, name of vessel, on-board cargo, port of destination and time of arrival together with the closest point of impact, their course over the ground and their speed, amongst other inane drivel. It is brilliant and I have become, I am ashamed to admit, an AIS geek.

We have developed a problem on board our little orange bateau. We have run out of onions! The situation has escalated quite dramatically and concerns are raised daily as to how our Mother Watch are supposed to cook spaghetti bolognese or sausage, mash and onion gravy without them. The situation became quite desperate last night when our wonderful pasta carbonara arrived on deck minus the said vegetable. At the same time we spotted a yacht closing our port bow.

However, with every culinary disaster comes a culinary delight. One of our crew has produced the most amazing bread, which has risen beautifully. I am sorry the same cannot be said for the second effort in the galley this morning. A rather interesting chocolate slab-shaped offering arrived on deck this afternoon masquerading, I understand, as chocolate brownies. Unconvinced of this we all tentatively took a piece, conscious not to offend the chef, and were stunned. Thank heavens looks can be deceiving!

A gentle day today with poled-out headsail and mainsail only – no kite. (*Now for those of you who still don't speak yacht let me explain. A poled-out headsail is very simple. With the boom holding the mainsail hanging out one side of the boat and the headsail hanging out on the other side of the boat being held there by a large yellow somewhat over-engineered scaffolding pole which we attach to the mast about fifteen feet above my head we present as much sail cloth to the wind as possible. With this sail pattern the wind, blowing from behind, is captured in all the sail cloth and propels us forward along our line towards our waiting rum. There – downwind sailing explained in a few easy lines – very simple!)*

We have rocketed along at ten knots speed over the ground with very little effort with the crew relaxed and chilled. We topped a wonderful two-hundred-mile day again today so all on board are very happy.

As night watches began one final treat for the day – dolphins! There were about fifteen of them playing on the bow, a wonderful way to end a lovely day.

Sunday 30 November

It is day eight and I have a dilemma.

Smell has to date played a huge part in sailing. As a new crew sets sail across an ocean, body and clothes cleaned in preparation, the whole boat smells of an interesting combination of Calvin Klein aftershave, Mr Muscle anti-bac, Bold 2-in-1 and Right Guard – all is well with the world. As the voyage proceeds the aroma gradually changes to something less sweet-smelling, but we are all in this together – and still, all is well with the world.

However, life is a little different on this boat, and last night I was instructed to arrange a laundry run. Each crew member was entitled to launder two items, and these were to be presented on the floor in front of the washing machine door in the laundry room just after breakfast.

I was thrown – clean clothes *and* clean body all on the same ocean crossing? Something was wrong. So the dilemma began – which items can I do without wearing again until I get home and which should I retrieve from the stinky laundry bag stuffed to the back of my clothes box?

Anyway, discussions began last night as to what constituted an item. One T-shirt was clear enough but how many pairs of Calvin Klein briefs were equivalent to one T-shirt? Worse – what was the ratio of thong to Calvin Klein briefs to boxer shorts? The dilemma was unimaginable in the cockpit and just to make things worse the black market was rife by dinner as one crew member said he did not wish to put anything in the machine! The crew shuffled through their storage boxes guestimating how many pairs of socks could justifiably fit into a two-item restriction. Me? As I was the one with the finger on the 'on' button on the washing machine, I managed to squeeze in one T-shirt, three thongs, two pairs of little trainer socks *and* a pair of shorts. Oh the power of the button!

Anyway, all was going well until someone – against the advice of the author I might add! – added five drying-up cloths and two towels to an already full laundry load, which quite frankly was a silly move. It completely overloaded the machine which after a huge five minutes ground to a halt. It flashed up Error Code 41 – which, when we consulted the manual, stated that we should call out the engineer. Unsurprisingly, I was not convinced that we would get someone to come this far so we levered open the door and deposited the soggy dirty laundry into the starboard shower tray and a crew member spent most of the morning on his hands and knees scrubbing our smalls – now that will teach the *male* guilty party to listen to a woman! Still by midday our sleek orange boat was looking disturbingly like a Chinese laundry, with all sorts hanging off the rails drying in the now scorching sun.

———

Sadly the wind died and the direction changed this evening, and our heavenly boat speed of nine and a half knots in the right direction was reduced drastically to five and half knots in the wrong direction. We put in a gybe just before bangers and mash arrived on deck so now at least one of those problems was solved. We are at least going in the right direction now – just very slowly.

Early to bed for me and my troops as I take the graveyard shift from midnight to 4 am.

Monday 1 December

Another scorcher. With the kite flying I am expecting to see a rather red-faced crew by the end of today. Today is American Education Day! Our two Americans are back in the galley as Mother Watch and whilst they were scratching around for ideas for toppings for our pizzas for lunch a discovery was made which required explanation. One of them appeared on deck and stated that whilst she was getting used to some of our English ways she was struggling with the concept of spotted dick.

So the day ticked on and the wind dropped. The kite came down as there simply wasn't enough wind to fill it let alone propel fifty tonnes in any direction. Our poled-out set-up was rigged into place with the yankee secured. This was helping us inch forward initially, but then the wind swung around and we found ourselves heading north. Not great! A gybe was executed with such precision that I smiled – truly a racing crew with speed and accuracy now. Once again, a drop in wind speed that we could ill afford. However, after lunch the crew was gathered on deck and a discussion ensued.

The result of this conversation was the sad decision to retire from the race, and at 1440 hours we notified the ARC race office, who confirmed our move to the cruising division of the crossing. The crew lowered the yankee and staysails, centred the main and cranked up the iron top sail (*the engine*). The crew sat with long faces, the silence was deafening. The reason for this decision was timing and a lack of wind. A difficult decision, but the statistics have given us no choice.

Tuesday 2 December

Cruising is supposed to be relaxing! We had a horrific night watch last night. At midnight my graveyard shift began with us arriving on deck sporting an array of night-time sailing wear from shorts and deck shoes to boots and jackets. We took over from a very quiet evening watch and enjoyed the first hour. From there on in it was mayhem! The wind dropped to a soul-destroying two knots and shifted round – so we dropped the yankee and staysail which had been lifted to give some extra drive. The flogging was very bad for the sails, and for the sleepy heads below decks. We inched our way through a very calm sea, no stars to light our way. Very eerie actually. With a wind shift the sails were re-hoisted to benefit from the now stormy conditions of eight knots of breeze! However, a sharp barometer drop set the alarm bells ringing and sent me scuttling off to the radar, which revealed an enormous rain pattern sitting just off our starboard bow. Unable to see this in the dark, we waited, and as the wind built and shifted 180 degrees we dropped the sails once again in time for the heavens to open! Man alive, I have not been that wet in my life – except in a bath of course.

Watch change brought weather change again with the winds dropping to two knots as we cleared the deck – typical – and I returned to a now damp bunk as the hatches had been left open!

So with dawn we scanned the horizon. The sea was stunning – flat, glassy and calm with a beautiful blue-grey hue, the sky thick with cloud and a sun trying its hardest to make its presence known.

Amongst other roles, I have been elected entertainments director – for reasons I have yet to discover – and so began my new job in earnest. 'I spy with my little eye something beginning with C'. After a few incredibly tenuous suggestions the answer 'cloud' rang out. Content in the knowledge that my entertaining was under way I disappeared off deck to check the weather. Entertainment plans for the afternoon were already afoot, with a movie and popcorn on the cards – oh the beauty of a large flat-screen television in the saloon!

Nail files, books, crossword puzzles and laundry all began to appear on deck throughout today – all new items on deck since we acquired our status of cruiser. A truly relaxed crew indeed.

Tea was skipped today in the presence of popcorn but supper arrived on time and the first watch took control of the deck – helming in a straight line was the order of the day. The rest of a rather frustrated crew went to bed, and sadly I could already see the signs of cabin fever setting in.

Wednesday 3 December

We have motored a total distance of three hundred and sixty-seven miles to date and cabin fever is well and truly setting in. However, relief came in the form of rain today. The downside to motoring on this little orange bateau is that we cannot run the water-maker so power showers have been put on hold to preserve the water in the tanks that we currently have for drinking only – until this afternoon that is, when the heavens opened and the entire crew belted up on deck in next to nothing armed with their shower gel and shampoo bottles.

As you can imagine – the rain started, we covered ourselves in the appropriate bubbles, and then the rain stopped. So there we stood looking at each other in fits of giggles ... and waited. Sure enough, not more than ten minutes passed and the heavens opened again, and as we huddled in a line under the mainsail, which was dumping extra water, we cleaned ourselves off and belted below, leaving one poor soul driving. Now that's what I call teamwork! With the boat now smelling like a tart's boudoir and with the appearance of a Turkish steam bath as the hatches have all been closed we continue our long motor towards St Lucia with very little hope of sailing again at this point – the computer weather files that we receive by email look dreadfully light and devoid of any wind. The wind hole that we are currently sitting in – the one that caused our downfall in the first place – is coming with us!

Thursday 4 December

Guess what! We are still motoring and it is still raining.

The crew were at their lowest ebb yet, with days of motoring already in the bag and more days still to come with no respite – so it was with great excitement this afternoon, when the new weather files were downloaded and then overlaid on the electronic charts, that we discovered wind – and from the right direction.

This meant the end of the engine, for a few hours at least, and sails! Hurray! The silence was wonderful after the drone of the engine – and it lasted for precisely one minute. We decided to take full advantage of the engine being off and turned the generator on instead to allow us to make fresh water to refill the one tank that we have used – safety first.

So with the engine off and the generator *and* water-maker now on we sailed our way across day twelve of our trip.

Friday 5 December

Today is Christmas Day. In Holland, at least – with a difference, however. The Dutch Santa Claus, Sinter Klaas, has a different story. He does not live in Lapland and arrive, sporting a red and white suit with white fluffy beard, on a sleigh pulled by reindeer. Nor does he have little elves with green hats to help him make the presents he delivers to all the good children in their stockings. Sinter Klaas arrives by boat from Spain, with a large white steed on board. He sports a cardinal's outfit with grey beard and his support crew are tiny men, not an elf in sight. The presents, which they have hand-made, are delivered together with personally written poems to the children who have left out, not stockings, but little shoes instead. Or so I'm told.

So that is Christmas, Dutch style. However, if you ask anyone in Spain where Sinter Klaas lives you will be met with blank faces. No-one has ever heard of him!

So Merry Christmas – or *Prettige Sinterklaas!* – to the Dutch sailors.

Saturday 6 December

Elation today! Finally, after some two thousand three hundred miles we have seen the much-coveted whale. After days of being confronted by Mary making wave motions with her left hand, apparently signifying a whale breaching, coupled with a ssssh-ing sound, which is apparently the sound a whale makes when it breaches, both done in the hope that it will bring the whales to the surface of our water, we have finally spotted two spouts followed by the required breaching whale! However, it was short-lived, presumably because the girls on board made such ridiculous squeaking noises of excitement that frankly only dogs (and whales?) could hear – which probably sent the whales in the opposite direction with their fins over the their ears. This excitement was missed by most of the boys on board, who have since decided that we have made the whole episode up.

The winds have filled in a little today, allowing us to motor sail, and we are making around nine knots over the ground with an arrival date of 9 December.

With the breakdown of the washing machine earlier in the week we have finally accepted the fact that we shall have to hand-wash our arrival T-shirts (which were also our departure T-shirts) rather than using the laundry.

Sunday 7 December

We were boarded last night – not by pirates but by a silly, somewhat lost egret who, after numerous attempts at joining the team on the deck finally made touchdown on the port quarter atop our race number. As my watch handed over the deck the little chap decided that there were more comfortable places to spend the trip so moved to the mainsheet. This presented the team with amusement for many hours, as each time the main-sheet bounced and tensioned the bird had to hold on for dear life for fear of being launched sky-high.

Today also brought wind. We had enough to sail this heavy beast (very briefly, it turned out again) so we hoisted the yankee and staysails, turned the engine off – silence – turned the genera-tor on – end of silence – turned the water-maker on and managed to get the whole crew through showers before the wind died and we turned the water-maker off, turned the generator off – silence – turned the engine back on – end of silence – and lowered the flogging foresails! A clean and, once again, frustrated crew. We motored for the rest of the day with the promise of winds of up to twenty knots from the weather files – but for once in their tiny little lives the stupid files are actually over-reading! Typical!

The heat was truly scorching today, which sent most of the crew to hide in the shade created on deck by the yellow sails. The boat looked like the land of the living dead. Heat exhaustion has taken hold.

Still we are one day and sixteen hours away from our rum.

Monday 8 December

Well what a day! We started wonderfully this morning with all the sails up and working hard for us. We were trucking along at ten knots speed over the ground in the direction of the bar in Rodney Bay, but by lunchtime not only were the foresails down but we had resorted to putting a reef in the mainsail in a desper-ate attempt to reduce the flogging. It is this flogging that causes expensive damage to both the sail cloth and the battens that run through the sail. This seemed to do the trick, and we motored along with this sail plan for some hours before the low-pressure system that had been moving north finally arrived with us and blew twenty knots – so like coiled springs the crew was up and hoisting every bit of canvas we could lay our hands on and finally, *finally*, silence fell on the boat – the engine went off, the music went off and we all just sat and enjoyed the power of sailing for one last blast before we cross the finish line in Rodney Bay tomorrow evening local time. Well, that is the estimated arrival time at present so long as the wind keeps blowing and we keep up at least nine knots.

So the end is in sight, and when not sailing the crew spent most of the day discussing their first drink. Beer or rum? Oh the dilemma! However, between now and that delightful drink there are a few chores to be done, to include re-inflating the huge fenders – which if handled correctly could take them all day. No point in rushing it now.

The heat has been debilitating again, and in between the lounging around on deck we noticed that we were joined by a large pod of dolphins who have come to play with us. They performed beautifully.

Tuesday 9 December

A busy day today. For me that is, not the crew. In an act of rebellion they have voted me in to do the final Mother Watch of the trip! Now I took to the seas to sail, and my ability in the galley is not well known, so on their heads be it.

I was joined by another crew member to help in this last Mother Watch. We began by rummaging through the cupboards and freezer and decided that we would treat the crew to bacon butties for lunch, a carrot cake for afternoon tea and a Thai green curry for supper. This seemed simple enough until I remembered that I had to make both the bread – two loaves – and the cake. An alarming look engulfed my face and I wandered off nonchalantly to ask strategic questions of the female contingent, trying unsuccessfully not to look desperate. The other mother was sent to clean the heads and bilges.

After numerous visits on deck to engage in cloak-and-dagger discussions regarding various aspects of whether I should follow the instructions on the cake packet, which stated that I should add olive oil to the carrot cake, or just ignore the instructions and do without I eventually appeared, resplendent in bikini top, shorts and an awful lot of flour, at the companionway sporting a grin from ear to ear. The oven was off, the bread loaves were out and cooling and looked fantastic and the cake – well, it was sitting on a plate looking suspiciously like a cake!

Later, at tea, as the crew tucked into my carrot cake there were no visible signs that they were devouring (at quite an alarming rate I might add) a cake that had been cooked twice – once the right way up at gas mark 8 for fifty minutes instead of the instructed gas mark 4 for fifty minutes (you can imagine the smell, and state the thing was in when I retrieved it from the oven – the saloon filled with smoke) and then again for a second time, upside down, in a desperate attempt to cook the still gooey inside of the cake after I had managed to prise it out of the cake tin and successfully cut off the burnt top and sides. Ignorance is bliss I think!

I am alarmed to note that not one fender has been blown up this afternoon. The race number remains on the wrong quarter of the boat and only three team T-shirts have made it to the drying stage on the guard rails. The crew, it appears, have taken this cruising lark to new heights and have decided to undertake none of the day's tasks, so they spent the day with their heads either in books, on pillows or attached to little white cables with music pumping into their ears. Again the deck looks like a scene from the land of the living dead in the relentless heat and between visits to the saloon I wandered past the chart table to check on our ETA and distance to finish in the hope that we might make rum o'clock this evening – local time, which is five hours behind GMT. Sadly we face another night at sea – but it does mean we can look forward to beer and Weetabix for breakfast!

After my prowess in the galley this afternoon I was banned

from the dinner preparations and my team-mate mother produced quite simply the best Thai green curry I have eaten. A grateful crew demolished their last supper at sea amid thoughts of a big fat steak and large glass (or bottle) of red to accompany it.

With a good twenty knots of wind blasting us ever closer to St Lucia most of the crew and I head off down below for one final snooze before chaos tomorrow.

Wednesday 10 December

Dawn arrival! Sporting our newly laundered team T-shirts and after a particularly hectic jostle with another two boats we tacked our way towards and then over the finish line in Rodney Bay to huge cheers. Sails were dropped and the deck was sorted out so that when we arrived in the marina we looked shipshape.

We were met by whoops from the yachts who had already completed the race. In amongst the din I could hear my name being called, and there on the pontoon was Gareth, a crew member from my transatlantic race team of last year, and his wife Ann, waving hysterically on the dockside. They have a home in St Lucia and were there for Christmas. It was wonderful to see them, and it made my arrival all the more special to be met by friendly faces.

Wednesday 17 December

After returning from the Caribbean this weekend I headed into BBC Radio Solent. They were hosting a party for all the 100 Lives participants to celebrate the end of their project. It was great to see the familiar faces, and there was a part of me today that was just a little bit sad that I was no longer going to be involved with the team on a regular basis.

On a personal level, I have enjoyed enormously sharing my story. I am certain that discussing my situation has helped me to acknowledge what I have been through and how I have fought and arrived at this place. I appear to have come out the other side – and I hope that I have helped others in my situation.

Thursday 1 January 2009

We arrived in the USA yesterday and spent last night, New Year's Eve, with good friends of ours, Marcus and Tatty, who live in New York at the moment. We had a wonderful evening, starting with drinks, followed by a fantastic meal in a great little French restaurant and finishing up with counting down the seconds to midnight while listening to a live band in the snow in Central Park. A truly memorable New Year's Eve.

Friday 2 January

Once again I was reminded today of just how many lives this horrible disease affects. We received news today that the sister of a friend of ours who was recently diagnosed with breast cancer has had a horrible reaction to her chemotherapy treatment. Having spoken to her soon after her diagnosis, and encouraging her to take whatever treatment was offered, I felt a certain sense of guilt having heard of the state she is in. Of course logic says that I could not have known how she would react to treatment (in fact not even the doctors can tell) but there isn't much about breast cancer that is logical.

Sunday 4 January

I went into BBC Radio Solent today to talk on a new subject. With the finish of their 100 Lives project and their year of interest in my life I was now invited in to discuss the subject of step-parents. I don't have any advice on being a good step-parent – hell, I don't know how to do it myself, but I do have my thoughts and views and ways in which I handle it. This is a new area for me but one I am now deeply involved with. I learn every day how to be a step-parent and how to handle not just the children but also Rich, their father. To add to this already quite daunting challenge the children live in the United States with their mother. We are incredibly fortunate in that we all get on tremendously well which makes our lives, and those of the children, much easier and happier. We also have the support of all her close family members in the USA who make our visits there happy for everyone. We work as a large team but I appreciate that this is unusual. We are incredibly lucky.

My task of learning to be a step-parent is made that much harder as I am not a parent myself. Learning to understand that one's actions and involvement in a small child's life is significant is tough in itself, but to do so with someone else's children provides a sharp learning curve. I take my lead from Rich and his responses to my actions. I love his children, Hannah, Dan and Nick, and fortunately they are receptive to me, my actions, my discipline and my love.

Sunday 26 April

I am an active individual, and earlier this year I set myself a new challenge. I did something very silly today and completed the London Marathon. One year late, as I originally applied to compete last year, but that turned out to be far too close to my reconstructive operation. However, with the blessing of my breast reconstruction surgeon I set off this morning to pound the streets of London.

It was amazing – as I stood on the start line of the world's most famous marathon with my puppies safely holstered for their biggest challenge to date my mind was buzzing – I had finally reached the start – a huge hurdle but I was there. I thought back over the past few months of training – the long runs around the area and when the weather was too horrid to bear taking to my running machine at home. Feeling like an oversized hamster I ran mile after mile and never left the house. Meanwhile, Diana, my sailing friend and marathon mate, had pounded the streets of Lymington and its environs in preparation.

Now, bobbing up and down on the spot to keep warm with thirty thousand other excitable runners, the atmosphere was electric. The voice that came over the loudspeaker was hysterical – 'could all animals please move to Pen 9' – now on the grounds that this was a race for human beings rather than our four-legged or feather friends, I assumed they meant costumed runners.

Anyway, we set off, heading out of the park. Dodging outstretched arms offering sweets, chocolate and fruit I pounded through the streets of London, mile after never-ending mile. Many were grabbing at the handfuls of Vaseline that were being offered by the St John's ambulance teams, but seeing as nipple rub is not a concern for me and my nose-less puppies I just kept running. It was a little soul-destroying at times, particularly being overtaken by a rhino. I wasn't having that, so I put on the pace and shot past him again. I suffered the same feelings when Scooby Doo and an emu ran past, and I dealt with them in much the same way at mile twenty-two.

I managed to have myself some nibbles en route, helping myself to the outstretched arms and their goodies, and after consuming numerous jelly babies, a Penguin (a chocolate bar – not an actual penguin!) and three cola bottles I finally crossed the line five and a half hours later. Not bad for an old girl, as my husband tells me! Diana and I finished within minutes of each other, which was fabulous. The legs were performing badly immediately after the run and now the feet have rebelled and refuse to go into shoes. On further inspection I note the odd blister and would advise anyone thinking of running a marathon not to do so in toe rings!

So there we have it. That's that challenge done. On to the next.

Sunday 10 May

I flew to the other side of the world today. In spite of my all-encompassing fear of flying, I boarded a plane bound for Madrid where I changed planes and endured a twelve-hour flight to Buenos Aires. After an all too brief stopover in a fabulously trendy hotel in the beating heart of this wild city I flew to Tierra del Fuego.

Ushuaia, the largest town on this island at the southern tip of South America, is very friendly and offers the most amazing views. Surrounded by snow-covered mountains, it takes the brunt of the winds from the Southern Ocean as they hurtle around Cape Horn. It is a truly magnificent place. We are not quite in the middle of nowhere, but we can see it from here – next stop Antarctica. (I never flew that far, unfortunately. I have a passion for penguins and desperately want to visit the emperor penguins, but clearly that will have to wait.)

I am down here teaching in what must be the world's most southerly classroom. I have joined *Pelagic Australis*, a superb ice-reinforced seventy-four-foot yacht weighing in at sixty tonnes, designed for expeditions in the high latitudes. She is amazing.

After their time with me in the classroom the students then leave Ushuaia and head out through the Beagle Channel, around Cape Horn and on to the Falklands bound for Cape Town. A wonderful adventure for them and I am very envious that I am unable to accept the offer to join them.

Tucked safely in my bed, I listen to the wind blowing the boat against the pontoon. Feeling very isolated, I note that the bottom of the world is a very long way down!

In conclusion

I have exited my cancer experience like a bullet out of a gun. Everything I do has to be done at one hundred miles an hour and I have to do it all now just in case I don't have much of a future left to do it in. I feel like an animal or a child that is worried to sit still just in case the cancer catches up with me. But as another year passes, so the belief in me changes. The further away I move from my diagnosis the more I begin to believe that I may have a future. I am beginning to believe in my strength and I am beginning, very slowly, to be a little less cancerphobic – not much, though, as recently I actively encouraged my medical team to approve a brain scan after experiencing headaches for a week. However, despite the headaches stopping and the huge knots suspected of causing the headaches in my neck and upper back being dissolved under the firm hands of a fabulous sports masseur, my medical team, who know me so well, agreed to allow the scan to take place regardless of a now obvious lack of symptoms. Needless to say they found nothing, but I was much happier.

I am told this neurosis will never go away but will diminish with time. It is a control thing. I have been put in charge of my body and my survival and I am not going to take any chances of messing that up and missing a symptom or sign. I am not going to let the same misdiagnosis fiasco happen again. It is tricky, bearing in mind the doctors cannot tell me exactly what I should be looking for as each person has different reactions and symptoms but could I please look out for them anyway. This does present something of a challenge.

True, my body is not what it was. It is a little tatty at the edges and definitely a different shape but it is the body I am in. I am now slowly reclaiming it and looking forward to doing things that make me feel whole again, rebuilding myself mentally now that the physical rebuild has been completed. Like many cancer survivors I feel stronger and fitter than before. Perhaps because I have had to fight for my life – and nothing can prepare you for that. I believe that when you have faced your own mortality, whether through accident or illness, life becomes a little more precious.

For me this is the end of an epic and unusual journey. I am almost home and dry and remain hopeful that I shall be a success story for the Royal South Hants Hospital, the Southampton General Hospital and the Salisbury District Hospital combined.

———

Has this whole experience changed me? Yes of course it has. It has challenged me in a way no other thing has, beyond my imagination. I would be a fool to think that something as serious as cancer would not change me.

Have I learnt anything? Yes of course I have. I have learnt about myself, life itself and everything else besides. Never have I been so glad to be as stubborn as I am though.

Do I live my life differently? Undoubtedly. I believe I am calmer and more tolerant than before. I think I would like to ask my friends and family how I have changed too, but am concerned that the answers may be just as intimidating as my experience with cancer itself.

What has this taught me? Well, there is always tremendous fallout from a life-changing or life-threatening event. It has enormous repercussions. For me, this life-changing event has taught me not to be afraid to try. I used to need to have all my ducks lined up in a row before I would try something, but now I will give anything a go, whenever, which is not always such a good thing! I won't just jump head-first into literally anything, but equally I can safely say that I am no longer afraid of trying. Fear can be a measure of your character, but it is immeasurable as an emotion.

When someone is diagnosed with cancer, or any other life-threatening disease, life screeches to a halt. You are sent on a detour, but for me it is these detours that have helped to remind me of who I am. I am beginning to view the whole breast cancer experience as lucky – not a word I would ever have associated with it before. It has been a positive experience in that I am learning to live in the present – because I don't know if I have a future.

I read back through my diary and find it difficult to believe that it is me I am reading about. It can be easy to forget sometimes the detail of the horror of it all, and yet part of me doesn't want to. My questions are many and varied. They are complicated, some are frightening, deep and challenging, and unfortunately some of their answers continue to elude me. There has been a mixed reaction to me since my diagnosis – both during the nightmare and as I come out the other side. People either see me as a ticking time bomb and step away waiting for it to explode again – because in their naivety they believe that no-one can actually beat breast cancer – or they help me. I am not trying to be a pioneer for all things breast cancer, I am just trying to live my life, a life I have fought for – and if, on the way, I can show that a diagnosis of breast cancer doesn't necessary mean the end of life as you know it then that is great. Those that offer help and support do so because they know it will help me to move on, to continue to rebuild my life, returning to normal and leaving it all behind.

A critical illness or injury has massive repercussions on a life, especially if you are freelance, as I am. Our life changed dramatically. We could not afford to go on honeymoon, our social life involves never going out because it costs money, the last time we had dinner together in a restaurant was during chemotherapy, we cannot afford to visit family and friends that live too far away because we cannot afford to get there. Life is a challenge, but at least we have one together.

I am saddened that I have lost some friends along the way, people who cannot understand or who probably find it quite hard to know what to say to someone in my position – although I will comment that it is much harder to *be* in my position. However, I have discovered much more.

I have learnt to be a little humble. I have spent a few weeks this summer skippering for the Ellen MacArthur Trust, a charity that inspires young people's cancer recovery through sailing. Each week I was faced with a group of smiling and excitable young people, each with incredible courage. Like me they have been through the nightmare of cancer and experienced the fear, the intense and sometimes brutal treatment that accompanies prolonged stays in hospital away from their families. They have not benefited from the joys of a normal childhood, and some have physical disabilities as a result of their cancer, and yet their strength and drive, energy and enthusiasm seem incredible from ones so young. I was truly moved, and spent the first evening of every week in a melancholy mood as I watched my new team for the week around the saloon table playing games, in awe of them. They were unperturbed by their situation and were quite simply overjoyed to be a part of this exciting adventure.

Without doubt my sailing helped me through my challenge. It was normal for me, but more importantly it took me as far away as possible from the treatment rooms and hospital wards that played such a huge part in my life. Out on the water it was as if the cancer was never happening. Sailing was a physical challenge that tested me and made me feel alive.

Life moves on and so must I, continuing to believe in myself and continuing to fight. Don't get me wrong, the wobbles still come and bite hard but my ability to reason with them is developing. I am never ashamed of my wobbles and my tears, they are a part of it all.

As a cancer survivor, to date at least, I want to forget it all. It is a horrific experience no matter how well the body handles the challenge, both physically and mentally, and to be forced to dwell on it and remember every detail is certainly not something

I want to do. I do acknowledge, however, that I still walk tentatively around the edges of a fatal disease – but I have no intention of sitting still and letting this blowfish catch me again. I have a life to live, a life I have earned.

———

Having had time to reflect on the past three emotional and challenging years, I now appreciate what a huge part my family and friends have played in my survival – and in helping me to find a way through this nightmare. One thing I have learned is never to hesitate to draw on loved ones when I find it hard to summon up the strength I need. Family and friends, in turn, should never underestimate the importance of the role they play. Never wonder what you can do to help. You may feel awkward and uncomfortable and not know what to say – but by just being there you are helping.

To all of Team Blowfish, named and unnamed, family, friends and colleagues – you will never know how much your support has meant to me. I appreciate the sacrifices and effort made for my benefit. I will never forget your support, love and commitment. Thank you.

Emma Pontin

Fifteen years ago Emma Pontin joined a law firm in the City of London and began an eight-year battle with the London Underground. Then, aged thirty-two and in search of an adventure, she crossed her first ocean and has never looked back. She is now an ocean-racing yacht skipper.

Just four years after her dramatic change of career, Emma was diagnosed with breast cancer whilst heading to the start line of a transatlantic yacht race. She returned home for a life-saving mastectomy but continued to skipper, race and instruct throughout her soul-destroying chemotherapy and radiotherapy treatment in a desperate bid to help her feel alive. And she returned to skipper the transatlantic yacht race exactly a year later – determined not to be beaten. She has since had a prophylactic mastectomy followed by bilateral reconstructive surgery. To date her battle with the cancer blowfish has been won.

Emma now has around 100,000 nautical miles tucked safely under her belt, including fifteen transatlantic crossings, three Fastnet races, one Newport to Bermuda race and the infamous Sydney to Hobart race. As a freelance skipper, she continues to enjoy life on the water, both racing and instructing. Her next big challenge will be breastcancerroundtheworld, a full circumnavigation with a novice team made up of breast-cancer survivors. With her big-boat sailing and team-building experience, together with a very personal understanding of breast cancer, she knows first-hand the strength that can be gained from sailing.

WALKING ON WATER
A voyage round Britain and through life

GEOFF HOLT

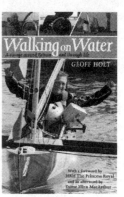

In 1984, at the age of 18, Geoff Holt broke his neck in a swimming accident. He was left paralysed, his promising career as a yachtsman at an end. 23 years later to the day, Geoff became the first quadriplegic yachtsman to sail single-handed around Great Britain. This is Geoff's story of his life before and after the accident: how he learned to live with his disability, how he achieved astonishing success in spite of it, how he rediscovered the sea and helped to promote sailing for disabled people – and how he conceived and completed the dangerous circumnavigation. With a foreword by HRH The Princess Royal.

> **'This is a story that will excite admiration from all sailors, disabled or otherwise'**
> Sir Robin Knox-Johnston

> **'Beautifully written and honest'**
> Dame Ellen MacArthur

Illustrated · ISBN 978-0-906266-09-7 pbk · Also available with companion DVD

ICE BEARS AND KOTICK

PETER WEBB

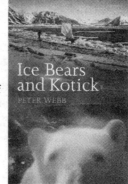

This is the story of an impossible boat journey that two men made for the fun of it. They rowed through pack ice and survived polar bears, starvation and capsize, and in doing so they completed the first circumnavigation of the Arctic island of Spitzbergen in an open rowing boat. Along the way they learned about themselves and about life, and experienced a wilderness that will most likely disappear before the century is out. This is a story for small-boat sailors, lovers of ice and snow, and anybody who knows anybody who wanted to run away to sea.

> **'An evocative tale of good, old-fashioned adventure amid one of the bleakest landscapes on earth ... vividly and thoughtfully written, an inspiration'**
> John Ridgway – first transatlantic oarsman

Illustrated · ISBN 978-0-906266-03-5 pbk

THE LAST VOYAGE OF
THE *LUCETTE*

DOUGLAS ROBERTSON

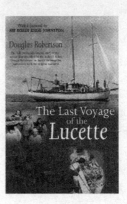

In their schooner *Lucette*, the Robertson family sailed from Falmouth in January 1971. 18 months out, in the middle of the Pacific, Lucette was holed by killer whales and sank. Four adults and two children survived the next 38 days adrift, first in a survival raft, then crammed into a 9-foot dinghy, before being rescued by a Japanese fishing vessel. This is a vivid and candid account of how they survived, but also of the delights, hardships, dangers, and the emotional highs and lows they experienced, both before and after the shipwreck. Douglas Robertson has taken his father's account, *Survive the Savage Sea*, as his starting point, but has also drawn upon his own memories of a life-changing experience.

> 'This adventure becomes more compelling in the context of his father having previously survived his ship being sunk by the Japanese during WW2; and Douglas, as a cadet in his first ship, surviving his second sinking in the Pacific'
> Royal Naval Sailing Association

With a foreword by Sir Robin Knox-Johnston · Illustrated · ISBN 0-9542750-8-X pbk

THE UNLIKELY VOYAGE
OF *JACK DE CROW*
A Mirror odyssey from north
Wales to the Black Sea

A J MACKINNON

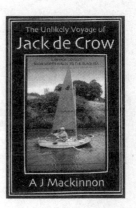

A couple of quiet weeks on the River Severn was the intention. 'Somehow things got out of hand,' writes A J Mackinnon. 'A year later I had reached Romania and was still going.' Equipped with his cheerful optimism and a pith helmet, this Odysseus in a Mirror dinghy takes you with him – 4,900 kilometres over salt and fresh water, through numerous trials and adventures. An epic voyage brilliantly told.

> 'This is a wonderful idea for a book – a series of ever bolder improvisations in the face of adversity, undertaken in praise of the spirit of adventure'
> *Times Literary Supplement*

> 'He must be considered the 'Captain Slocum' of the inland waterways of Europe. If you want a good read, go and buy this book'
> *Royal Naval Sailing Association Journal*

Illustrated with maps and line drawings by the author · ISBN 0-9538180-5-5 pbk